FAT, FAT, GET RID OF THAT

The Focus Diet

FAT, FAT, GET RID OF THAT

The Focus Diet

John T. Dedousis M.D.

iUniverse, Inc.

New York Bloomington Shanghai

Fat, Fat, Get Rid of That
The Focus Diet

iUniverse books may be ordered through booksellers or by contacting:

iUniverse
1663 Liberty Drive
Bloomington, IN 47403
www.iuniverse.com
1-800-Authors (1-800-288-4677)

Because of the dynamic nature of the Internet, any Web addresses or links contained in this book may have changed since publication and may no longer be valid.

You should not undertake any diet/exercise regimen recommended in this book before consulting your personal physician. Neither the author nor the publisher shall be responsible or liable for any loss or damage allegedly arising as a consequence of your use or application of any information or suggestions contained in this book.

ISBN: 978-0-595-47778-4 (pbk)
ISBN: 978-0-595-71465-0 (cloth)
ISBN: 978-0-595-60099-1 (ebk)

Printed in the United States of America

To my wife Elaine, my true love from the day we met
Alexis and Jaime, You're a part of me, and I'm a part of you.
My parents, who made sure I had the opportunities.
My sister Lisa, its always an adventure.

CONTENTS

Introduction

Over the past nineteen years of practicing medicine, I have had the unfortunate experience of watching many of my patients become larger and larger. With this increase in size, came an increase in the amount of medication they were taking. First, the cholesterol numbers would elevate, then came the high blood pressure. Soon diabetes would often kick in, as these diseases were correlated with the weight gain. As these ramifications of their weight would start, I would always do the right thing by telling them to go on a diet and put them on the proper medication. For some reason many of these people could not find success. Some would try this diet or that diet, others would "try to eat right," while the rest could not get the inspiration. As the time went on some of these people would develop all three of the above. Since these diseases are stepping stones, I soon was watching the drug companies getting wealthier as these people would soon move on to the secondary diseases that hypertension, diabetes, and high cholesterol would lead them. The heart attacks, strokes, kidney failure, loss of limbs, joint replacements and so on are all secondary from one underlying cause, our love for the wrong kind of foods. You don't need to be a doctor to see this phenomenon. Look at your friends and family, as I am sure if you are a typical American household, there are people in that group who are overweight, with some obese. If they are in the over forty club, they are probably on at least one pill. When I started being a doctor this was subtle, however over the past few years, despite all these advertised diets, obesity has become painfully obvious. This trend is not just occurring in America, it is also spreading to other parts of the world.

When I see an obese forty year old who comes for their physical and for the first time in their life has high blood pressure, it usually follows the same pattern. It is like the road ahead is carved out. Pills number one, two, three and more soon come. Arthritis of the limbs along with back, hip and knee pain. I know in many of these cases this is an avoidable future.

It was with this understanding that I decided to learn about the intricacies of weight loss. First it was some medical courses, then textbooks, analyzing studies, followed by incorporating these into my practice of medicine. As I worked with my patients I began to analyze all of them not just from a weight perspective, but also from a psychological perspective. I noticed that anyone can diet and lose a few pounds, but the ones who were truly successful in not just losing, but keeping it off had certain characteristics and perspectives. I learned that it was not just about diet. It was about real change in thinking, attitude and lifestyle. It was about recreation of self. As these people's lives were changed, the other added benefit that occurred, was the removal of medication by me. In many, as their bodies transformed back to health, there was no longer a need for that diabetic, hypertension or cholesterol pill. As weight loss goals were accomplished, patients on insulin up to 100 units a day were gradually taken off till it was no longer needed.

This book is not going to show you some fad diet because as you probably have learned they do not last. Every diet out there will help you lose some weight temporarily, but why do we gain it all back?

This book is going to show you

1) What is going on to cause this epidemic

2) Why some people lose easier then others

3) Finding your reasons and develop inspiration

4) Rules and regulations to weight loss

5) Your new dietary lifestyle

6) The truth about exercise and activity

7) Teaching you focus points to help with recreation of self and way of thinking needed to achieve continued success.

This book is going to give you the ability to not only lose the weight, but more importantly to think differently and create a lifestyle for you to keep it off and live healthier. <u>As you read this book you will see focus points in bold. Answer these points at minimum in your mind, but preferably in writing in the focus section at the end of the book. From this point on, I also want you to keep a food diary.</u> Buy a cheap notebook and write down every single thing that you eat and drink and how it was cooked (fried, grilled etc). Later in this book the value of this food diary will be explained in more detail.

CHAPTER 1

▼

WHAT THE HELL IS GOING ON?

Why is the population getting so big? Sixty percent of the population in the United States is now considered overweight, and 35 percent are considered obese. Obesity seems to be everywhere. Go into a room full of people and look around, and the truth will become obvious. Most of us are either overweight or obese. Why is this occurring? What is the impact on us? Why is obesity more prominent in minorities? Why are people who make less money more prone to obesity? Most importantly, why is obesity approaching 15 percent in our children? These are painstaking truths that are occurring in the United States.

Before we discuss these topics, we should have an understanding as to the definition of the words overweight and obesity. There are a few ways to define the terms, but a simple common way is to use a measurement called defined Body Mass Index or BMI for short. This is your weight in kilograms, divided by your height in meters squared. This is complicated, so to find it easier use the chart that follows this paragraph. To figure your BMI, find your height in inches on the top, and your weight on the left side. Once this is done, find where they intersect for your number. For example, if you are 66 inches tall and weigh 210 pounds, you have a BMI of 34. Between 19 and 24 is considered your ideal body weight. Below 19, is considered underweight. If you are between 26 and 29, you are overweight.

HOW TO DETERMINE BMI
(Height in inches)

Weight (Pounds)	60	61	62	63	64	65	66	67	68	69	70	71	72	73	74	75
100	20	19	18	18	17	17	16	16	15	15	14	14	14	13	13	12
105	21	20	19	19	18	17	17	16	16	16	15	15	14	14	13	13
110	21	21	20	19	19	18	18	17	17	16	16	15	15	15	14	14
115	22	22	21	20	20	19	19	18	17	17	17	16	16	15	15	14
120	23	23	22	21	21	20	19	19	18	18	17	17	16	16	15	15
125	24	24	23	22	21	21	20	20	19	18	18	17	17	16	16	16
130	25	25	24	23	22	22	21	20	20	19	19	1	18	17	17	16
135	26	26	25	24	23	22	22	21	21	20	19	19	18	18	17	17
140	27	26	26	25	24	23	23	22	21	21	20	20	19	18	18	17
145	28	27	27	26	25	24	23	23	22	21	21	20	20	19	19	18
150	29	28	27	27	26	25	24	23	23	22	22	21	20	20	19	19
155	30	29	28	27	27	26	25	24	24	23	22	22	21	20	20	19
160	31	30	29	28	27	27	26	25	24	24	23	22	22	21	21	20
165	32	31	30	29	28	27	27	26	25	24	24	23	22	22	21	21
170	33	32	31	30	29	28	27	27	26	25	24	24	23	22	22	21
175	34	33	32	31	30	29	28	27	27	26	25	24	24	23	22	22
180	35	34	33	32	31	30	29	28	27	27	26	25	24	24	23	22
185	36	35	34	33	32	31	30	29	28	27	27	26	25	24	24	23
190	27	36	35	34	33	32	31	30	29	28	27	26	26	25	24	24
195	38	37	36	35	33	32	31	31	30	29	28	27	26	26	25	24
200	39	38	37	35	34	33	32	31	30	30	29	28	27	26	26	25
205	40	39	37	36	35	34	33	32	31	30	29	29	28	27	26	26
210	41	40	38	37	36	35	34	33	32	31	30	29	28	28	27	26
215	42	41	39	38	37	36	35	34	33	32	31	30	29	28	28	27
220	43	42	40	39	38	37	36	34	33	32	32	31	30	29	28	27
225	44	43	41	40	39	37	36	35	34	33	32	31	31	30	29	28
230	45	43	42	41	39	38	37	36	35	34	33	32	31	30	30	29
235	46	44	43	42	40	39	38	37	36	35	34	33	32	31	30	29
240	47	45	44	43	41	40	39	38	36	35	34	33	33	32	31	30
245	48	46	45	43	42	41	40	38	37	36	35	34	33	32	31	31
250	49	47	46	44	43	42	40	39	38	37	36	35	34	33	32	31
255	50	48	47	45	44	42	41	40	39	38	37	36	35	34	33	32
260	51	49	48	46	45	43	42	41	40	38	37	36	35	34	33	32
265	52	50	48	47	44	43	42	40	39	38	37	36	35	34	34	33
270	53	51	49	48	46	45	44	42	41	40	39	38	37	36	35	34
275	54	52	50	47	47	46	44	43	42	41	39	38	37	36	35	34
280	55	53	51	50	48	47	45	44	43	41	40	39	38	37	36	35
285	56	54	52	50	49	47	46	45	43	42	41	40	39	38	37	36
290	57	55	53	51	50	48	47	45	44	43	42	40	39	38	37	36
295	58	56	54	52	51	49	48	46	45	44	42	41	40	39	38	37
300	59	57	55	53	5	50	48	47	46	44	43	42	41	40	39	37
305	60	58	56	54	52	51	49	48	46	45	44	43	41	40	39	38
310	61	59	57	55	53	52	50	49	47	46	44	43	42	41	40	39
315	62	60	58	56	54	52	51	49	48	47	45	44	43	42	40	39
320	62	60	59	57	55	53	52	50	49	47	46	45	43	42	41	40

A BMI over 30 is considered obese, which is then broken into three categories. A measurement between 30 and 34 is mild obesity. Between 35 and 39 is moderate obesity, and any level over 40 is considered extreme obesity.

Now that you understand the term, let's focus on its importance and discuss some of those important questions raised.

This rapid increase in obesity didn't happen overnight. Obesity has been steadily climbing since the 1970s at a pace of 50 percent per decade. In the past 10 years BMI levels over 40, which is extreme obesity, have doubled. The important thing to remember is this rapid rise in obesity has been occurring as Americans pour hundreds of millions of dollars into diet plans. Jennie Craig, Nutrisystem, Weight Watchers, Atkins, South Beach, Infomercials, and Herbal Products, are just some of the diets being consumed by the public. Think of all the books on weight loss in the bookstores. This is such big business that some of these companies are traded on stock exchanges as public companies. For as good as these products are, we keep right on gaining weight. We are now at the point where we are not only paying for the weight loss, we are now also paying for our failure to lose. The monetary effects of our obesity will cost Americans one hundred billion dollars a year in consequences. Heart disease not only in the form of heart attacks but also as congestive heart failure is becoming prominent. Your heart is a pump designed to deliver blood throughout the body. When your weight increases, the heart must work harder to pump to those additional pounds. Over time it simply gives out. Look at it this way, if I asked you to flex the bicep muscle on your arm fifty times, you could probably do it without a problem. If I handed you thirty pounds in dumbbell weights, and asked you to do the same thing, chances are the muscle would give out and you would fail. Well your heart is the same. It is a muscle just like the one in your arm. Give it too much weight and it can't do the job. The cost of medications for the treatment of hypertension is escalating. With this disease the incidence of stroke increases. Since obesity causes obstruction to your airway while lying down, sleep apnea is now being seen in large numbers of the population.

Our obesity is causing additional weight on our knees, hips, and back, causing arthritis at an early age. Think about it, these joints are the foundation of our body, much like the foundation of your home. Building a three story building over a foundation designed to be one story, would cause problems with the support and structure. The same goes for your back, hips and knees. If you are 6 feet tall, these joints were designed to hold 180 pounds. When you are 260 pounds at this height, the added weight pushes down on this foundation. This causes grinding, with wear and tear and degeneration, as the cushions designed to protect these areas are obliterated. Once this occurs the pain starts. If you are mildly overweight and can't grasp this concept, consider strapping an additional 30 pounds around your waistline and see how your back and hips feel after a short while. I guarantee it will hurt.

Diabetes is growing at an alarming rate, as 80 to 90 percent of all new diabetics are obese. The sudden growth in this disease is coming from our enormous intake of processed carbohydrates causing our pancreas, which makes insulin, to burn out. In addition, our increase in body fat, and decrease in the utilization of our muscle mass, is causing insulin resistance. This means our body isn't able to use the insulin we are making, as our body has developed a resistance to it. As this occurs our body tries to make even more insulin which causes increased fat production in our bodies. This syndrome then leads to hypertension, and elevated triglycerides. When you have the above with a waist size over 40 inches in a male, or 35 in a female, you have what is known as Syndrome X. This is the beginning of many bad things to come, as multiple medications for diabetes, high blood pressure and elevated lipids start showering upon you with heart attack, stroke and kidney disease looming out there in the horizon.

The cost of these diseases with medications, physician care, hospitalizations and so on is astronomical. Drug companies see this and salivate, as they develop new expensive drugs that this population will be dependant on taking. Yet with all the money we spend on weight loss, one diet plan after another, why can't we accomplish our goal?

The simple
answer is:

1) Wrong foods and too much food.

2) Less movement.

3) Complacency and always looking for an easier way.

Wrong Foods: There are some of us in the population who consume very large quantities of food all the time, and by that very nature they will gain weight. However in my practice I find that is not the norm, except in the very extreme obese patients. What I do find is most of us just eat incorrectly.

God designed our bodies to eat the things he created for us. Natural foods such as grains, fruits, vegetables, and animals were put on this planet for us to survive. It has always been man's nature to utilize these foods in a natural way. Doing this, our bodies remained the way we were meant to be. It was not until the technology era when we began to process our food, tampering with nature so to say, that this obesity began. If you are older then 45, think back when you were young. Growing up during that era, eating out was not the norm. We primarily ate fruits, grains and vegetables. We packed a healthy lunch. Dinner, cooked by our mom, was a balanced meal with some meat, vegetables and potato or rice. Over the past 20 to 30 years this has steadily changed. The restaurant business is now the cornerstone of the American economy as it now accounts for five hundred billion in sales and represents 4 percent of our gross domestic product.

Years ago we would get up and have our cereal or oatmeal with our coffee. We would then go off to work with our packed lunch consisting of a sandwich and some fruit. At night we had our balanced dinner, and later if watching a movie, some popcorn. Today we run out of the house in the morning so we can stand on the Starbucks or Dunkin Donuts line to pay for a 380 calorie 10 grams of fat banana frapachino with a 320 calorie 62 grams of carbohydrates bagel, combined with another 200 calories of cream cheese containing 17 grams fat. We then go off to work picking at high carb high fat processed snacks through out the day that one of our coworkers brought in for everybody. We will then go out for lunch which will be a 220 calorie 16 grams of fat quarter pound burger with 400 calorie 20 grams of fat French fries and a 110 calorie 30 grams of carbohydrate soda. At dinner time like many of us do frequently, we might eat at a restaurant or get take out where we will consume bread and butter, chicken parmesan with pasta on the side and a salad covered in ranch dressing. This adds up to around a thousand calories, fifty grams of fat and around a hundred grams of carbohydrates. This is excluding an appetizer and dessert, which can often double the meal in calories, carbo-hydrates and fats. It is no surprise that in areas where restaurants are more prevalent, there are higher rates of obesity. Think about it, as there is more competition restaurants are more inclined to offer more food for your money. In addition as there are more eateries in an area, the quality of the food is better, making it more condu-cive to dining out. In high population areas look around, there are fast food places everywhere. Burger King, McDonalds, Taco Bell, Kentucky Fried Chicken, the list goes on and on. All designed to make it easier for you to just pick up your food, rather then cook it. It is also inexpensive, resulting in our poorer communities using this form of eating as the norm. The problem with this form of eating is that it has replaced the balanced diet with a diet high in carbohydrates mixed with fat. Americans mix the two together over and over. We take a potato (carbohydrate) and cook it in oil (fat) to make French fries or potato chips. Use mayonnaise (fat) with the potato, to make potato salad or mix it with butter (fat) and milk to make mashed potatoes. We take dough (carbohydrate) cook it in oil (fat), inject it with jelly and sprinkle on sugar (carbohydrates) and call it a donut. By mixing Cheese (fat) and dough (carbohydrate) we make pizza and cheese snacks. We mix Cream (fat) and sugar (carbohydrates) to make ice cream, or add some cocoa to make chocolate. We take a healthy chicken cutlet, dip it in milk and egg (carbs and fat) then in breadcrumbs (more carbs) cook it in oil (more fat), then put cheese (more fat) on top and bake it in the oven. When done put it in a 400 calorie Italian roll with tomato sauce (more carbs), and call it a chicken parmesan sandwich.

When dining in restaurants, we gravitate toward the choices higher in fat without realizing the impact to our waistline. Two people going to a steakhouse, can seemingly order the same thing, yet when analyzed can be dramatically different. Both order a steak, potato and a salad. Person one gets the rib eye, mashed potatoes, and blue cheese dressing on his salad. Person two gets the filet mignon, baked potato with some margarine and vinaigrette dressing on the salad. Person one consumed somewhere in the range of 150 grams of fat while person two consumed about 35 grams of fat. The bill was the same, but much different health consequences.

Our snack food choices have gone from fruit to processed food. Entire aisles in supermarkets are dedicated to products rich in carbohydrates and fat. These products are also loaded with artificial chemicals and colors used as preservatives that our body was never designed to eat. Boxed donuts, cookies, cakes, chips, candy, chocolate, the list goes on and on with carbs and fat combined in a high caloric chemical mix designed to make us gain weight. Go into your kitchen closet and read some of these labels. They contain ingredients, half of which you can't even pronounce. A laundry list of things not meant to be in our bodies, are contained in these processed snack foods. In addition to the probable carcinogenic effects on all of us, many of these chemicals may cause leaky gut syndrome. This occurs as these chemicals inflame the intestinal wall making it more permeable to toxins, microbes and waste products. This makes us prone to water retention, bloating and fatigue. As these chemicals go through our bodies, they go through our lymphatic system causing them to be over-loaded, helping to produce the cellulite many of us have. Unfortunately, it is not just in our processed food. Many of our vegetables are sprayed with pesticides, and the meat we ingest contains hormones. If you look in the supermarkets, many people are now trying to avoid this by buying organic food products.

While all of this is going on, we are now living in what I call the super size era. Think back when you were young when the size of a bottle of coke was 8 ounces. If you look at soft drink websites now, a child size soda is 12 ounces. Most bottles now are 16 to 20 ounces in size. A regular cup of coffee no longer exists, as it is now a tall, grande or venti. Look at the muffins in the donut shops as they overflow around the wrappers. Go into a fast food restaurant and for a little more your order can increase in size. Why not for an extra 50 cents? Restau-rants do this to boost profits on low cost items like

French fries and soda. The cost to the restaurant may be only 15 cents while they get the customer to spend another 50 cents on something they wouldn't have ordered without the incentive. Replicate this many times and it comes out to be a lot of money. Replicate this many times and it also adds up to a lot of calories.

Less movement: While our eating habits have been changing over the years, so has our level of activity. Years ago, children coming home from school would leave the house to play. As a young boy, I would play football, basketball or baseball for hours on end. Whatever was played, body movement and the burning of calories was involved. Adults mowed their lawns and actually would walk to places as often as they drove. There was still a decent size in the manufacturing sector in the United States, as many jobs required physical labor and activity.

The technological wave over the past 20 to 30 years has changed all of this. Almost all of our manufacturing is now done overseas in countries like China and India. The little that is left for the most part is automated, which involves much less physical activity. Most jobs in this country today do not require the physical labors of years past.

The children today also have less activity. Although there are children who play sports, it is usually more organized for fixed periods of time. In many schools, gym is not mandatory every semester. Due to safety concerns and lawsuits, many school grounds are closed. Children now come home and sit at the computer sending text messages to their friends, or play video games for hours.

More Americans are now living in the suburbs then ever before. There we are now more prone to get in the car to drive to get a quart of milk as we think about that gym membership we never have the time to use. We have become so lazy we don't even get out of the car at the fast food restaurants anymore. Pull up and you will see a line around the building at the drive through window, while inside you can walk right up to the counter.

As we are eating more and moving less we have one more exponential factor. We are stressed and not sleeping well. As a nation, America is loaded with all forms of stress. This is very prominent in big cities where the pace is usually faster and more hectic. Long work hours, two job households, paying the bills, fulfilling our children's needs, keeping them out of trouble, amongst many other things, not only cause us to eat incorrectly and exercise less, but also raises cortisol levels in our bodies. When this occurs, our blood pressure elevates and increases storage of body fat. This occurs because the increased levels of cortisol make the fat cells in our belly become more resistant to losing weight.

As we live our stressful lives, many of us are not sleeping correctly. This becomes obvious when we see all the sleep remedies advertised in the marketplace. When we deprive ourselves from sleep, growth hormone, which is produced during these hours, decreases in our bodies. When the levels of this hormone drops, there is an increase in fat deposition in your body making it very difficult to lose weight and very easy to gain. This cycle feeds on itself, as the bigger you become the greater the chance of developing obstructive sleep apnea. This is a syndrome that primarily affects the obese, where the excess weight causes obstruction in the pharyngeal area. During sleep hours this obstruction causes snoring and changes to your breathing which are dangerous. People who have symptoms of snoring excessively, sleep disruption, and daytime tiredness should have this investigated by their doctor, as this will not only impede your weight loss but can be dangerous to your health and needs to be corrected. As you can see each thing I just mentioned forms links to a chain that is difficult to break.

Complacency: As a nation of technology, we are continually looking for an easy way to lose the weight. This fad diet, that herbal pill, or some prescription medication, are the attempted quick solutions to try to solve our problems. We are all searching for that easier way so at the end of the day we can still eat that ice cream that we love, or those chips that we crave. Unfortunately like most things in life, we are learning the hard way, as America is beginning to learn the consequences of these habits. There is a saying by an unknown author that says; "there is no elevator for success, you have to take the stairs." This saying holds true with most things in life, however the trip doesn't always have to be miserable. Learning the way to eating correctly can be done without horrible sacrifice if your mindset and focus is in the correct mode.

So in a nutshell

Eating too many wrong foods
+
Lack of Activity
+
Stress
+
Lack of Sleep
+
Complacency
=
Obesity
Time for a lifestyle change!

CHAPTER 2

▼

THE CALORIE GAME

When people discuss weight loss, it is not uncommon to hear how a certain food has too many calories, or all they have to do is eat less calories to lose the weight. Few however truly understand how the body takes in and uses these calories. If you ask the average person what a pound is, the answer would be 16 ounces. Ask someone who understands weight loss and the answer is about 3,500 calories. A calorie is a measurement of energy, and for a person to gain or lose one pound, this is how many calories must be eaten or burned additionally to gain or lose that pound. Everybody has a metabolic rate that is unique. Think of it in terms of cars. Every car has a different engine, and gas is the fuel for all. Some cars burn gas faster and get less mileage per gallon and some engines burn fuel slowly and get better mileage. Humans are very similar as our metabolism is our engine and food is our gasoline. People who have a fast metabolism will burn these calories faster and lose weight easier. People who have a slower metabolism find it more difficult to lose weight.

Physicians who practice weight loss management will usually test your metabolic rate by doing a test called calorimetry. This exam helps evaluate what a person's metabolism is like. Doing this can help determine how many calories your body needs each day to keep your weight the same, or what is required to gain or lose. Lets suppose on testing your body, it has a resting metabolic rate of 1,800 calories. This would mean if you did nothing all day you would burn that amount of calories. Therefore, if you ate 1800 calories your weight would stay the same. Most people have some level of activity throughout their day. Unfortunately, in today's world it is minimal. So let's add a paltry 300 calories for going to our car, sitting at our desks, and walking to the vending machine. Therefore, if you consume 2100 calories, your weight will stay the same. Suppose you decide you are going to diet and eat 350 less calories each day. Since one pound is 3,500 calories, divide this by 350 and it will take you 10 days to lose a pound. Conversely, if you were to eat an additional 350 calories each day, in 10 days you will have gained a pound.

If you decide to work out, the same rules apply. Depending on your metabolic rate, the average person burns about 200 calories for these 30 minutes of basic exercise. Correct, about 3 oreo cookies for your 30 minutes of hard work. Divide 3,500 by 200 and you will lose a pound about every 17 days. Exercise however over time will help increase your metabolic rate, and burn calories easier, but for now you are not in that place.

Activity is another way to burn calories. Take the stairs instead of the elevator. Choose a parking space further away at the mall. Cleaning your house, doing your garden, mowing your lawn, will burn calories. In fact increasing your daily activities can burn 500 to 700 calories a day.

Lets show the power of additive effect. Suppose we ate less, exercised, and did more each day. 350 + 200 + 600 = 1,150 calories. Divide 3500 by this number and you will lose a pound every 3 days. This number is not too shabby. As you will learn later, what you eat will also help influence your weight loss. However the concept here is you need all of the elements to have success. **Dietary change**, **exercise** and **activity** are all necessary aspects in your new lifestyle if you wish to lose weight on a consistent basis and stay healthy.

Chapter 3

▼

The Steps To Success

Something inspired you to pick up this book. Maybe the name caught your eye or a friend recommended it. Maybe your doctor just started you on medication for the first time for hypertension, diabetes or high cholesterol. It might be because lately your back, knees or hips have been hurting. Possibly you just feel it is time to make changes in your life, lose a few pounds and start living a healthy lifestyle. Inspiration can come from many sources, but for someone to be successful at something, it is usually a necessary part of the plan.

Nobody in New Jersey just gets into a car and drives to Boston. There is usually a reason for the trip such as a business meeting, vacation weekend, or seeing family. It is that purpose that makes you get in the car and drive for all those hours. Once the reason is established, you have to believe that you will be able to have the time and ability to get there. Unless you have been there many times, you don't just get in a car and start driving without direction, hoping you will arrive there. You begin the process of learning the directions. You will use a map, maybe go online, ask someone who has been there, or call the hotel, but there is a learning process. At that point you will set a date and at that time you will take action and begin your journey. To make this trip you will have to sacrifice some time and effort to get there. While traveling, you may make a wrong turn or get off at a wrong exit. If you are dedicated with a good enough reason for the trip, and truly focused on getting there, you will find your way back to the correct road and eventually make it to Boston to accomplish your goal. While there, hopefully you will enjoy your visit for its duration.

What does a trip to Boston have to do with losing weight? The answer is everything. In order to lose weight, there has to be a reason or inspiration. The people who just say "I have to knock off this weight," never do so with any long lasting success, as they have not defined a reason or inspiration to do so. Once you have your reasons, you need to know your goal. It should be clear and defined. You have to say I am going to be this weight by that date. At that point you need to learn how to get there. You need to follow a plan with directions on how to achieve your goal. A roadmap for your trip, that is a plan you will follow without variation. It should be clear, concise and leading to your goal. While you are on this trip called weight loss to a destination called X pounds, you will make wrong turns by consuming food you should not have eaten. When this occurs, you can either go back to your old ways, or you can regain your focus and find your way back to the correct road to complete your journey. Once you arrive, you do not want to turn back and go home right away. You want to enjoy your destination to its fullest. You want to take every opportunity to make the most of the time and effort put into the trip. Like most trips, you will be happy you went. The same will go with your new dietary lifestyle. When you have accomplished your goal, you should be able to enjoy the fruits of your efforts and continue to do so life long.

Everything in life follows these principles. It doesn't matter whether you are going to Boston, losing weight, becoming a doctor, or pursuing any particular career. It's all the same the same formula.

1) **Reason or Inspiration**

2) **Goal or Destination**

3) **Belief you can do it**

4) **Roadmap on how to get there**

5) **Taking Action**

6) **Some sacrifice for the better good**

7) **Going through Mistakes**

8) **Staying focused and persevering**

9) **Attain the final result**

10) **Focus on continued success**

These steps are the keys to success. To become a doctor, I first needed the inspiration. I set my goal and believed I could attain it. I investigated what it required and then took action and attended medical school. I went through some difficult times but I stayed focused and eventually became a physician. Like with all good things in life, sacrifices had to be made along the way. While many of my friends were going to parties during college, I was studying. When they were working after college making an income, I was a broke medical student for many years. I stayed focused, and like most things in life that require sacrifice, it was all worth it, as success has its sweet rewards.

Weight loss and lifestyle change are no different. There will be some nights where your friends will be eating ice cream in front of you and at that point some choices will need to be made. If you stay focused and choose wisely, I promise you the reward at the end will all be worth it.

This book is designed to educate you on how to diet and lose weight. Unlike every other fad diet on the market, it will also take you through each of the steps to help you keep your focus and make sure you have long lasting success. Following this program, you will develop a new outlook on your health and achieve a new lifestyle with life long results.

CHAPTER 4

▼

INSPIRATION

It's time to figure out why you want to lose weight. There is an obvious dissatisfaction with something or you wouldn't have bought this book. People who are dissatisfied tend to do one of three things.

1) They wallow in it, become depressed, continuing on a destructive path. During this time they make one excuse after another as to why change can't occur.

2) They pretend it doesn't exist laughing it off, saying this is the way they are. When it comes to food their outlook is they want to enjoy life and this is their way of doing so. They tell other people that they will have to accept them. Unfortunately, people do have sterotypes against obese people, and there are so many health hazards that later will make life difficult.

3) They decide to make real change in their lives. They use the dissatisfaction and turn it to their advantage. They use it as the driving force to turn things around. Time and time again we have all read or heard about multimillionaires who came from very poor backgrounds. To these people it was either change or live a life of poverty. The same holds true with those who have finally hit the point of ultimate dissatisfaction with their weight. At that point dissatisfaction can be used as the incentive and inspiration to make a change.

Maybe you have been dissatisfied but have been procrastinating. I'm going to start after the holidays, after vacation, or after the summer. Next week has probably turned into many pounds more then what you have wanted, and now you realize the costs, as you see the consequences of your weight. Maybe you are doing this now because you have no choice. When someone does something because they have to and not because they want to, they will only be good for a short while. They will then revert back to old familiar ways when whatever forceful pressure has eased. If you don't want to, eventually you will begin the process of sabotaging yourself. You will begin to use every excuse in the book. It was boring, the food was no good, it was too hard to follow, etc, etc. This process also occurs in people afraid of success.

In order to lose weight, keep it off, and live a healthy lifestyle you need to want these things. Since you want them for the long term, you need to evaluate your situation no differently than any other thing you would commit to for a long period of time. You need to know all the costs and benefits. You need to write down what the cost has been to your body. What will the cost be to your body in the future if you do not change? What will this change in life cost you? How will this change in lifestyle benefit your body?

Let's look at some examples of each topic for you to get an idea of what I mean.

Has your body paid any price for the weight that you are at the current time? If you are still early in your life and mildly overweight, the answer might be it has not. If you are obese, or older, maybe you have begun not being able to do things that you used to do. For example, playing sports and climbing stairs without gasping for breath may be things you were able to do easily in the past. Maybe your back, hips or knees are beginning to hurt. Maybe you have begun to develop some of the health risks associated with obesity, such as hypertension, high cholesterol, fatty liver disease or obstructive sleep apnea. Hopefully you haven't yet developed the secondary effects of the above diseases. Heart attack, stroke, cirrhosis, kidney disease and arthritis to name a few are all secondary to the above with obesity often times the root. If you are there, you are on multiple expensive medications.

Is getting out of bed harder? Are you tired and exhausted after work with no energy? Do you sit on the couch during this time only able to watch shows on television? Has your weight affected your ability in developing relationships? Has it affected your self-esteem or made you feel less attractive when you approach someone of interest? Maybe you have been overlooked for a job or a promotion at work, as whether you like it or not, there is discrimination in the workplace.

Have you noticed obesity affecting your children? Are they becoming overweight like you? Do they hold a similar future?

Focus point #1) Write down the cost you have paid for your weight.

Lets go into the future as you age. Lets go 10 and 20 years ahead. First of all if you are over 50 and over 300 pounds and go forward 20 years, chances are you won't be alive. Ask yourself how many 300 hundred pound people do you know over 70 years old. Hopefully, this is food for thought. If this is you, change must occur now. However, let's move forward for most people. Your knees, hips and back are now so badly degenerated that you are using a walker and probably need joint replacement. Unfortunately, you have too many medical problems making the surgery unsafe. You are on a multitude of medications. Your children are now adults and if they had the same eating habits, you are watching them walk down the same path you have traveled.

Focus point #2) Write down the price you will pay without change.

Now that you have some thoughts as to what the cost of your weight is, lets explore the cost of change. If you are obese, chances are you have been eating incorrectly. The biggest sacrifice will be a change in the way you have been taught to eat. You need to change your perception about what food is good. When we say a particular food is good, we usually mean in its taste, which lasts for that brief moment. Since all of us always answer the most important thing in our lives is our health, we need to think of good food as food that is good for our health for the long term. This will mean a sacrifice with the foods that we perceive as good. Processed foods and snacks like ice cream, chocolate, boxed donuts, and chips will need to go. Fatty meats like spareribs, cold cuts, and fried foods will need to be a thing of the past.

You will need to learn to move your body. You will start to exercise on a regular basis. You will stop sitting on the couch, and start to take on activities that require body movement.

With everything good in life, there is usually sacrifice. Nothing in life is a free ride. You can't just party in school and expect to have a great career when it is over. It usually requires some hard work and studying, and in the end it pays off. The same concept is applicable to your weight. You can't be healthy and eat whatever you want. Some sacrifice will pay you big rewards and when you begin to reap them, you will not want to eat those foods you thought you would miss so much. All good things in life have a cost, but it is the end result that matters. Success in life does not come from laziness, but from desire and work. All things in life adhere to these principles.

So now you have the price tag on changing your life. In short, it is avoidance of certain foods and adding exercise and increased activity to your daily life. Hopefully, as you continue to learn the specifics and move forward it will be an enjoyable ride.

Focus point #3) Write down the price you will pay to change.

In addition to knowing the above, you need to have some expectation as to how these changes will affect you. In the beginning of your first week or two you will feel the discomfort of sacrifice as you will talk about how you miss ice cream or whatever food you crave. Whenever my patients return after their first week and I ask how they are doing, the initial response is always "doc I don't want to lie, I really miss my _____". They get on the scale and see the positive results but they don't feel the results. In a few weeks however, they notice that they are feeling better. They begin to have more energy and can do more. The best is when I begin to remove medication. As six pills a day becomes five, then four and so on they develop a feeling of happiness and satisfaction with themselves. Some of my single patients tell me they are beginning to go out and date more. My married patients with children tell me they are doing more activities, and are noticing the kids losing excess weight as their eating habits are changing.

Let's bring this out 10 to 20 years since you have changed your lifestyle. If you were 300 pounds over the age of 50, and lost the weight by changing your ways, you are alive and actively enjoying life. For the rest of the world you have slighted the pharmaceutical industry by keeping billions of dollars in revenues they would have received from people like you. Instead of that money going to them, it was used for other good things in life like vacations, a car, or retirement. You age gracefully without the pain that obesity would have caused. You can call these years the golden years and not the rusty years as I hear so many people call them. Your children are now adults, healthier due to the way you taught them to eat. They are not on a multitude of medications, instead they exercise and are vibrant.

It's time to stop looking at the quick pleasure you receive eating whatever unhealthy food you enjoy, and start looking at the ultimate benefits of changing your life. It's time to see the big picture from a distance. It's time to get a handle on your self and take action.

Focus point # 4) Write down what you will ultimately achieve by being your desired weight.

Stop the procrastination
Stop making excuses
Stop laughing it off
Stop sabotaging yourself

Hoping, wishing and saying," I want to lose the weight this year," will not get you where you want to be. Only desire and devotion to a new way of life will get you to your destination.

Focus on the long term benefits.
Focus on the belief you can make a change.
Focus on your health.

I understand that you may feel some resistance in writing out these exercises however, I also know you want to lose that weight and be a healthy person. You may only be mildly overweight at this point in your life and your goal is to lose a few pounds. For most people it is much more and writing things down will allow you to visualize what you are thinking and doing. It serves as a reminder on a daily basis as to why you need to change, and how you are going to do it. Soon I will teach you how to lose weight, but to truly keep it off you have to know the reason to start your journey. This is your opportunity to understand yourself and make the change necessary for success.

CHAPTER 5

▼

GOAL OR DESTINATION

Now that you have your inspiration to change your life, it's time to set your goals. When a person does goal setting, timelines must be put in place in order for them to be effective. In the beginning of the book there was a body mass index chart. This is a good place to start if you are not sure what your weight should be. A correct weight should be under the 25 level. I keep mine at 24 on the dot. The inaccuracy of the BMI chart is in the muscle mass. When a person has a great deal of muscle through exercise, it weighs more then fat. Your weight therefore will be more, however it is all muscle, which is a good thing. Many times as my patients are approaching their goal weight, the pounds stop going down, but the inches on their body are showing a dramatic loss. This is because they are at the point where the exercise is really beginning to kick in and real muscle is forming. So if you are all muscle, a slightly higher BMI may be acceptable.

You need to pick a weight that makes you comfortable. Often times when I show people their proper BMI of 24, they tell me they have never been that weight and it is too low for them. I always hear that they are "big boned". No obese person has small bones. Understand, just because you have never seen that weight, doesn't mean you shouldn't be that weight. Nothing is unrealistic, if that is what you want. However, if you feel the weight should be a slightly higher number go to a BMI of 25 or 26 but not higher. Find this number and set it in stone by writing it down. By doing this process, it will keep you focused on your goal weight.

Next you will need to set your timeline. Take the weight you are now and subtract your desired weight. This will be the amount you need to lose.

For example, you are 190 pounds and your goal is 150 pounds. You therefore need to lose 40 pounds. Each person will lose weight at a different pace. This will depend on your metabolism, how much excess water weight you have, caloric intake, exercise, activity, underlying medical problems, and naturally compliance with the proper food. If you have a great deal of water weight you will lose a lot in your first week or two, however this will revert to a normal pace subsequently. A person who eats properly and follows the basic rules of exercise and activity can lose up to 3 pounds per week, but 2 pounds per week is a realistic number to use. If you want to be conservative you can use 1 1/2 pounds per week. If you are losing less, you are either doing something wrong or have something that needs to be medically evaluated. Some people are very aggressive, especially with exercise and can see dramatic results. To some a couple pounds a week is not dramatic enough. Remember this is not a fad diet, where you will be starving yourself, then gain it back later. This is a change in your lifestyle and thinking. Using 2 pounds per week as a guide, take the amount of weight you need to lose and divide it by this number. Forty pounds divided by 2 and you get 20 weeks. So within 5 months you should be at your desired weight. If it happens at a different pace fine, but at least you have a set goal. Remember the trip to Boston. You might hit traffic, or it could be clear sailing, but at least you want to set an approximate time of arrival that you can kind of count on. Mark off on your calendar the date you expect to reach goal. When you start your weight loss protocol, write down in advance the weight you expect to be at the end of each week. This will help you keep your focus, as each week you will see if you are where you are supposed to be. Once again if you are saying this exercise is a waste of time, I am telling you it is not. Any successful person will tell you they start projects by writing things down, creating a draft and format for their plans and goals.

Focus point #5) Write down your goal weight and date of expectation.

CHAPTER 6

▼

THE ROADMAP, OVERVIEW OF FOODS

Here is the chapter that is going to give you a roadmap to the foods you can and cannot eat while trying to lose weight. It is important to realize not all foods on the avoid list will be forever. There are certain foods that are natural and will be allowed once you reach your goal weight. At that point you will be in a maintenance mode for your weight. In this chapter you will begin the process of learning how to lose weight, therefore certain foods will not be allowed until goal. So here are the rules for losing weight.

Rule # 1) Lots of Water

Every diet tells you this concept and there are good reasons. Water assists in digestion and absorption of food, and helps with the excretion of waste by helping to avoid constipation while your eating habits change. Water also acts as a natural appetite suppressant. When a person hasn't eaten in a while, the stomach contracts and fills with acid. When this occurs, the brain sends a signal to your body that you are hungry and to do something to fill the stomach. Since water has no calories, when you drink it, you are filling and distending your stomach without calories. This will decrease the hunger mechanism, as your brain will interpret that there is something in it. Will it completely satisfy you? The answer is no, however remember we are working on the additive affect. Distending the stomach to some degree will mean you will want to eat less. This is why it is especially important to drink water before a meal. On any given day, you should consume about two quarts of water. Spreading it out throughout the day is important, but you should try to drink 8 ounces prior to eating to curb your hunger.

Rule # 2) Only Smart Carbohydrates

There is no question that processed carbohydrates is a major factor with obesity in the world today. Over the past twenty years or so as we have used technology to artificially process our food, the population has been steadily increasing in weight. Soda and sugar based beverages, particularly with high fructose corn syrup, are a concentrated high calorie food. Anytime you ingest a processed sugar, within a few hours you are triggering hunger within your body that will cause you to eat more. This is because when you eat a high sugar or carbohydrate food or beverage, it will cause a rapid rise in your blood sugar. When this occurs your brain will read your sugar going up and tell your pancreas to rapidly make insulin to lower this level back to normal. As insulin is released rapidly, within a few hours your sugar will drop quickly. When your sugar starts the rapid descent, your brain reads that the numbers are dropping faster then usual and will then sound out a hunger alarm for you to eat again. During this time you might feel shaky, weak, sweaty or just hungry. This cycle is especially prevalent with processed carbohydrates as these are prone to cause rapid swings in your sugar levels. Natural carbohydrates such as grains, fruits and vegetables are absorbed differently without the rapid swings in blood glucose levels seen with processed sugars.

The diets that tell you to eat no carbohydrates are not healthy either. Yes, you will lose weight on them but do so by putting your body in an unnatural state called ketosis. When this occurs, there is a breakdown of fat into energy, which burns calories but puts a stress on your body. When this is done for extended periods it can be dangerous, especially for diabetics.

Foods that we traditionally call starches are for the most part your potatoes, rice and pastas. These are natural fillers that different cultures use to fill the plate. The problem with many of these is we like to add fat in their preparation. In their natural state, they are fine to eat in limited amounts while maintaining your weight. When you are trying to lose weight, they impede the process, making it harder to accomplish your goal.

Juices are natural but you are concentrating the calories of many pieces of fruit into one glass and this is not conducive to weight loss.

So while trying to lose weight in your new diet there will be

   1) **No Sugar**

   2) **No Flour**

   3) **No Juice**

   4) **No Rice**

   5) **No Potatoes**

   6) **No Pasta**

Cereals are acceptable if they are bran, grain or oat in nature. No sugar type kids cereals and no rice or corn cereals. Oatmeal is a soluble fiber that keeps your hunger in control and therefore is a great breakfast.

Vegetables are a natural healthy carbohydrate and are encouraged. While trying to lose weight, it is probably better to avoid the starchy types such as corn, carrots, peas, beets and as above potatoes. All other forms of vegetables are highly recommended for you to get in the habit of eating on a regular basis. These should be used in high quantity, as they are water based, low in carbohydrates and fat, and filling to the stomach.

Breads that contain flour, such as white bread, are to be avoided. Natural bread made from grains such as wheat and multigrain types are healthy and should be used. While trying to lose weight, it is mandatory to use regular sliced bread or wraps of these types and not rolls or bagels. Incorporating light brands of breads will allow you to have 2 slices for the calories of one. Muffins should not be used while trying to lose weight.

Fruit is God's natural sugar to satisfy our sweet tooth. Unfortunately, man wasn't satisfied with this and had to create all kinds of processed sweetened foods. It's time to get back to basics and start eating fruit again. While we are in weight loss mode it should be two portions per day. A portion is defined as one piece of fruit like an apple or an orange. It can also be a cup of chopped fruit. I encourage eating bulky fruits like apples, pears, and cantaloupe. They are high in fiber, take some time and effort to eat and are quite filling. Small fruits like grapes are consumed quickly and do not leave you with a feeling of satisfaction.

Rule #3) Limit Your Fats.

One would think that this is a simple concept, however the food industry and fad diets have attempted to put a twist on this. Some diets would have you believe that the problem of obesity is not in the fat but in the carbohydrates consumed. As these diets became popular, many people were eating meats and other foods high in fat content. As the public became educated that this was unhealthy, another false concept was created. The food industry began to tell people foods like French fries prepared with oil low in trans fats were healthy. This is not exactly the truth.

I'm not going to bore you with a long lecture on fats, but it's important to understand basic facts so you can learn how to use fats in your dietary habits.

Saturated fats and trans fats are bad for your health as they raise blood cholesterol. Hydrogenated fats are the same. Foods most likely to have these fats are foods from animals like meat, egg yolks, milks, cream, butter, and certain plant oils like palm and coconut. Foods like cookies, cakes, French fries and donuts are usually made with these fats. Consider what the fat looks like left in the pan after you cook meat such as bacon. This is the exact grease that enters your body. Think of the arteries of your body as the pipes of your house. If you knew that you had some clogged pipes in your house, would you dump bacon grease down the drain of your kitchen sink? The answer is no because you know soon enough you would be calling the plumber. The same goes when you eat foods high in fats particularly the saturated type. These fats go into the pipes of your body called arteries, and when there is a build up, you're calling your doctor for that balloon angioplasty and stent to open up that pipe. This is only if you were lucky enough to catch it before it completely clogged an artery causing a heart attack or stroke.

Polyunsaturated fats and monounsaturated fats are healthier. Polyunsaturated fats tend to help lower your cholesterol and reduce these deposits on artery walls. These come from certain plant oils. The polyunsaturated type from safflower, sesame, soy, corn and sunflower oils. Nuts and seeds also are included in this group. Monounsaturated also come from plant oils such as olive, canola, and peanut oils.

When you have a healthy weight, oils and foods that have some polyunsaturated fats are fine in moderation. When you are trying to lose weight, all fats need to be limited to a marked degree. Although the polyunsaturated type may be healthier, all fats contain more then twice the amount of calories then either protein or carbohydrates. Look at the information on the side of the olive oil container. The amount of <u>calories is 120 per tablespoon.</u> Think about how many tablespoons you splashed on that salad you thought was helping you lose weight.

So with this new lifestyle of losing weight, the rules on fats will be: All meat eaten will be low in fat. Meat is basically composed of protein and fat, and the fat composition varies depending on the type of animal and the cut of meat. It is time to eat meats that are low in fat so from now on you will **eat lots of turkey, chicken, veal and fish.** If you are a person who needs beef on occasion, it must be a **high quality beef as in filet mignon or sirloin with limited use.** This type of meat is seen in the supermarket and should say ninety percent fat free on the label. Beef should be limited to once a week. **Try to keep away from pork**, because for the most part this is a fatty animal. There are some center cuts that are ok for rare occasional use. The meats mentioned are what most people eat, however frequently I am asked about other types. Meat such as venison would be an example of something brought up by my patients. Looking this information up online in the world today is easy, however I like keeping things simple. If the animal is large and stands around all day grazing and eating with little activity like a cow or pig, chances are it has a lot of fat. If the animal is one that is active and runs around in the woods and eats nothing but plants like a deer or rabbit, chances are it is low in fat. Like people, other animals that eat right and exercise don't have a lot of fat.

You will not eat processed meats. What is processed meat? This is any food where they take all the leftover parts of an animal, grind them up, add fillers and chemicals and shove it in some kind of casing. Examples of these are hot dogs, sausage, and kielbasa. Most cold cuts like bologna, liverwurst, salami and pepperoni to name a few are in this list that goes on and on. **The exceptions to this rule are the high quality processed turkey and chicken.** I am referring to your quality turkey sausage and burgers, etc. You will know, because it will say on the package that it is ninety percent fat free. If you see this, it is ok to eat. In the deli section of the supermarket turkey breast, chicken breast, and ninety plus percent fat free low sodium ham are ok for sandwiches on your multigrain or whole wheat bread.

Dairy products must say low fat, as most dairy in its natural state is high in fat. Low fat milk in limited amounts and a low fat cottage cheese is fine. If you enjoy eggs, the fat is in the yolk. The white is all protein and healthy for you, therefore egg whites are fine, or you can have eggbeaters. **Cheese and butter are not to be eaten,** as these are solid blocks of fat. **Oils will also not be allowed since these are liquid fat. Nuts** also have a high fat content. **Keep away from these products.** I am aware that there are fat free cheeses and ice creams, however I want to break the habit of eating this type of food and get you to start developing tastes for different foods that are healthy.

Rule # 4) No Carbs mixed with Fats.

This is the most dangerous combination, the old one two punch. This combination is usually found in most of our snack foods, and is a key ingredient in the recipe for obesity. So from now on **No Cake, Pastries, Cookies, Doughnuts, Chips, Cheese snacks, Chocolate, or Ice cream. The list is endless as you go down the snack food aisle. Basically if it comes in a bag or box with fancy colors, you shouldn't be eating it.**

Rule # 5) No Salt.

The human body keeps a constant ratio of salt to water. When you are dieting or anytime you take in extra water, in order to keep a constant balance, your body will excrete this excess water in your urine. However if you take in extra salt, your body will hold in the water to keep that steady balance. When this occurs you will retain water weight. So stay away from the saltshaker and foods traditionally high in salt like canned foods and fast foods.

Rule # 6) Drink Healthy

We talked about the benefits of pure natural water however I understand not everybody wants to drink only water all day and night. Diet ice teas particularly green teas, sugar free lemonade, or club soda with lemon or lime are fine to use. There are the many flavored waters now available in stores. Coffee and teas are ok, but remember they have a diuretic effect and will make you urinate more. I'm not a big fan of diet soda as it is a little harsh on the stomach and usually loaded with artificial colors and chemicals, however from a weight loss perspective they are acceptable. **You cannot drink regular soda, beer, wine, or hard liquor, while trying to lose weight.** If you are at an occasional party and must have a drink get one of the ultralite beers on the market and nurse it throughout the evening.

Rule # 7) Use healthy Condiments

It is time to learn how to cook without the fat and begin to use spices and herbs to prepare your meals. On your salads, do not use oil or cream dressings, **use only low calorie, low fat dressings**. There are so many on the market now that finding them is not difficult.

Mayonnaise in its regular state is a definite no, however the light forms are not unreasonable. One tablespoon is about 4.5 grams of fat, so if you use it, make it a rare occasion, and go easy because it will add up.

The following list is a group of condiments I want you to begin to use when preparing your food. These are usually low in calories and fat. Many of these can be used as marinades when cooking your meals. Learn to use this list as opposed to the following unhealthy list.

Healthy List of Condiments

Mustard	Salsa
Ketchup	Barbeque Sauce
Hot and Tabasco sauces	Sesame
Lime or Lemon Juice	Cocktail Sauce
Meat marinades and seasonings	Peppercorns
Crushed Tomatoes	Horseradish and Mustard
Guava paste	Garlic
Relish	Spices

Herbs	Balsamic Vinaigrette
Teriyaki	Soy Sauce
Relish	Balsamic Vinegars
Dried Tomatoes	Worcestershire Sauce
Peppers	Margarines (limited)
Butter Sprays	

Learn how to cook with these items. Be careful as some may contain elevated sodium content, however you must learn to garnish your food with methods that limit fats.

Unhealthy List of Condiments

Mayonnaise	Horseradish Sauce
Butter	Tarter Sauce
Creamy salad dressings	Cheese or Cheese Sauces
Sour Cream	Oils

Get out of the habit of using condiments from this unhealthy list and your body will thank you by taking off pounds.

Meat gravy tends to be made from the fat drippings and flour, however there are some fat free types on the market. If flour is used however it is still on the no list.

Rule # 8) Use Sugar Substitutes

Since sugar is a definite no, many people complain that they need their coffee or tea sweetened or that they need a sweet snack on occasion. I realize that sugar substitutes are artificial and not natural, however like everything in life you have to weigh the benefits and risks of choices. As I stated earlier in the book, sugar adds on calories and creates swings in the glucose levels of your body. Sugar substitutes have no calories and help you achieve your weight loss goals. Like anything in life if used in excess, they are probably not good for you. Use them in moderation only when necessary. The three most common on the market are aspartame (Equal), dextrose (Splenda), and saccharin (Sweet n Low). My own personal preference is the dextrose, however you may decide for yourself.

There are some snacks with sugar substitutes such as diet gelatin, puddings and yogurts. These are very low in calories and will help you achieve your goals. I would prefer you learn to break the sweet tooth habit and go natural, however I understand that certain times we desire something sweet to satisfy our taste buds. So you can use these sweeteners judiciously.

Rule # 9) Cook Healthy.

As I mentioned earlier, it is important to prepare your food using healthy condiments. **When you cook your meals you can bake, broil, roast, boil, steam, barbeque or grill. You will never fry your food in oil, lard, animal fat or butter. If you fry something, it will be with all natural cooking spray, but never fry meat as it will sit in it's own fat while cooking.** An example of this kind of spray is PAM Organic.

Rule # 10) Always eat snacks or desserts that will help you with your goal.

The one snack that you must begin to enjoy is fruit. This is the snack God gave you naturally to satisfy your sweet tooth. As you start your new eating habits, I want you to **eat two to three pieces of fruit every day.** Yogurt, that is sugar free and fat free, is another healthy snack, as well as the sugar free gelatin and puddings mentioned earlier. I want you ice cream lovers to break this habit even in its diet form. I find that later on you will drift back to the regular ice cream, which is very fattening and unhealthy. Lately, there have been many new snack bars on the market. Some are healthy and some are not. Those that are, make a wonderful snack when you have reached your goal weight and are in a maintenance phase. Until then, I want you to stick to the above.

Remember these rules. They are put in a simplified format at the end of the book as a reference or for you, or to put on your refrigerator for quick review.

In the introduction of this book, I asked you to keep a food diary. I want you to now circle everything in that book that breaks the above rules. If you ate fried food, circle it. Cookies and cake, circle it. Chances are there are a lot of circles in your book. These foods circled are the ones that packed on the weight and got you to where you are right now. As you move forward, the next chapter will lay out your meals. I want you to continue with your food diary. Include everything you eat and drink and how it was prepared especially for the first eight weeks.

A lot of people think this exercise is stupid, however it allows you to visualize what you are doing. If you did poorly on a particular week and didn't lose weight, you can review what you ate each day and see if it violated any of the above rules and how often it occurred. The same holds true if you did particularly well one week, you can go back and see which foods work well for you. Doing this simple exercise will allow you to see the impact certain foods have on your body, and how you respond to them.

Focus point # 6) Focus on memorizing the 10 rules of weight loss and using your diary to attain your new lifestyle.

CHAPTER 7

▼

THE ROADMAP, YOUR MEALS

Now that you are familiar with the overview, lets break this down into meal form to get an idea as to how your day should be. As you eat your meals, **remember not to overindulge yourself. Eat until you are reasonably content and then step away from the table.**

Another important aspect in your meal plan is to **make sure that you do not eat the same things everyday.** Many times in my office, people bring me in their food diary and on it I will see grilled chicken every night for dinner and turkey wrap everyday for lunch. They will have lost weight that week, however sooner or later they will be sick of the repetition and go back to their old ways. When doing this, you are temporarily dieting, and eventually will gain the weight lost back again. It is crucially important that this is a new lifestyle that will continue. To attain this goal, learn different ways to prepare the foods mentioned in these chapters. Take an interest in your new lifestyle. Since this will be a long lasting commitment, buy a good recipe book that teaches you how to cook in a light fashion. Start preparing the foods you eat with your own hands. Doing these things will guarantee that it was prepared correctly, save a lot of money, and teach you a whole new way of eating.

Breakfast Anyone of these would be appropriate.

Cereal. A half to three quarters of a cup of a cereal that is an oat, wheat or grain type. Examples of these are Cheerios, Wheaties, All Bran, Fiber One, etc. Remember no corn, rice or sugar cereals. Your cereal can be eaten with no more then 3/4 cup of low fat or skim milk. This can be used up to three times a week.

Oatmeal. This is probably the healthiest of breakfasts. It is all oats, no fat, made with boiled water and a dash of low fat milk if desired. This can be used as often as you like.

Eggbeaters or Egg Whites. No more then the equivalent of two eggs made in a pan with PAM spray. Inside of your omelet can be vegetables such as peppers and onions if you wish. On the side can be a slice of a low calorie whole wheat or multigrain toast with a small amount of margarine. This should not exceed 3 times per week.

Low fat, low carb yogurt. There are many kinds of yogurt on the market. There are the regular yogurts, low fat yogurts, and the low carb yogurts. I want you to buy the kind that is both low in carbs and fats. An example of this would be dannon light and fit. This is the ideal breakfast for someone who doesn't regularly eat this meal or have time in the morning to prepare something. This can also be used as much as you like.

Low Fat Cottage Cheese. This is another healthy breakfast for those on the go with little time. Low in carbs and fat and high in protein, this choice makes sense as often as you wish.

Whole wheat, or multigrain English muffin. This is acceptable with a small amount of low fat margarine. This can be used up to twice a week.

Any of the above choices are acceptable to eat for breakfast. Remember no rolls, muffins (even whole wheat), croissants, or regular eggs. No pancakes, waffles or doughnuts. All of the above breakfasts should range between 120 to 200 calories and are prepared in a nonfattening way. They are all quick and easy so they can be done at home in a manner of minutes. For those who are not breakfast people, this meal is necessary.

Lunch. Any of these would be appropriate.

The good old fashioned sandwich. When preparing a sandwich remember that most cold cuts are fatty so you need to be selective.

Good choices would be:	Turkey Breast
	Chicken Breast
	Low Fat Ham
	Tuna in water

These sandwiches should not be overstuffed with the meat, and should be on a low calorie whole wheat or multigrain sliced bread. Use a healthy condiment if needed. If you use light mayonnaise, make sure it is less then a tablespoon.

A Wrap. These are becoming more and more popular and can be bought at many restaurants and even corner stores.

Good choices would be:	Grilled Chicken	Grilled Shrimp
	Turkey	Grilled Vegetables

The wrap itself should be wheat, as opposed to traditional flour wraps.

A Salad. This could be a regular salad or one with as many vegetables as you like. No cheeses or fattening cold cuts should be added. Grilled chicken, grilled shrimp or tuna can be on top if desired. It is imperative that a low fat, low calorie dressing be used. Caesar dressing is not low in fat unless it is specifically stated on the label.

Soup. This is an excellent choice for lunch. Vegetable and chicken soups are good examples. No cream or pasta soups. Here is a novel idea, do like mom use to do. Cut up a bunch of vegetables and chicken and make a fresh pot of soup. Put it in containers and freeze to use when needed.

Dinner.

This is not as difficult as you think. The most important point is remembering to prepare it in a healthy manner.

The Meat. This has to be low in fat or you will defeat the purpose of the diet.

The following are good choices: Chicken

Veal

Turkey

Fish

Filet Mignon or Sirloin
Steak (once per week)

The turkey used can be processed if it states on the package that it is low in fat. Turkey sausage and burgers are examples of this.

The fish can be any type, even shellfish like lobster and shrimp are acceptable, however you can't dip them in butter or tarter sauce. You can use the diet butter sprays and cocktail sauce if you desire.

The steak must be either a sirloin cut or preferably a filet mignon. It should not be larger then the hand of an average person.

Remember you cannot fry the above. You can roast, grill, barbeque, broil, boil or bake. Do not use butter or any fatty garnishing when preparing the dinner.

Vegetables. In addition to the meat, there should be 2 vegetables or preferably a vegetable and a salad. When preparing the vegetables, remember to prepare them in a nonfattening way. No oils, butter or cheeses are to be used.

No Starch. This is a crucial aspect to the weight loss process. That means as long as you are trying to take weight off there will be **No pasta, potatoes, rice or bread at the dinner table.** This will change when you have gotten to goal and wish now to only maintain your weight. Until then this is a price you have to pay.
Snacks. These are important, as they are a very big reason why we gain so much weight. We love our chips, nachos and doughnuts. Snacks can be a very dangerous thing when used incorrectly. However when used properly, they can be an effective tool in helping you to lose those pounds. The reason for this is the next focus point, which is one of the most important aspects of losing weight.

Focus point # 7) Never be hungry when you sit down to eat the main meal.

This concept is important, because if you are starving when it is time to eat, you have already set yourself up to eat too much. This is where the snacks will help, as you will eat six times a day to accomplish your weight loss. You read correctly, six times a day.

When you wake up in the morning, you will eat one of the breakfasts listed above. Lets just say for example it is the early morning. As the day progresses you will be sipping your water. By late morning, as lunch approaches, you are getting a little hungry. At that time you will have a piece of **fruit.** As you get closer to noon you will have a full glass of water. You now have put fruit and water in your stomach, and as lunchtime comes around, your sandwich will be more than adequate to satisfy you.

As the day continues with you sipping your water, come 4 to 5 in the afternoon, the early hunger starts in preparation for your 6 o'clock dinner. At that point, probably on your way home from work, you will have another piece of fruit. When you arrive home you will have another glass of water, then you will have your salad just prior to dinner. See what you have done, you have just filled your stomach with fruit, water and salad. This is filling your stomach with minimal calories. As you sit down to eat the main meal, you will not have that starving feeling so many people have at the dinner table, so your piece of meat and vegetables will be more then satisfying.

As you are watching the television at night, if you are hungry, you can have some **diet gelatin** an example of this is diet Jell-O**, diet pudding, low fat low carb yogurt, vegetable sticks** dipped in a low fat low calorie dressing if desired, or another piece of **fruit** if you are not a diabetic.

When I talk about fruit remember it is one piece. One apple, pear or whatever, it is not a big fruit salad. It is always fresh, and not in some kind of syrup. It should preferably be a bulky fruit like and apple or pear as they are filling, as opposed to grapes, which seem to never satisfy. If you use a small fruit it should be a portion, which is a small cups worth.

Those of you who are diabetic always ask about the fruit in their diet. My response is that you will be limiting the starches and other sugars in your diet during this process. Second, fruit is absorbed differently then processed sugars. Third, if you are diabetic make sure you limit yourself to two portions per day and not the possible three stated above. Make sure you stick to the portion concept of one piece. If your sugar does elevate, discuss this with your doctor. I have found in my practice that my diabetic patients sugar drops as they do this diet and the medicine decreases over time.

Can you see how snacking can help your weight loss as opposed to making you gain? By using this method, you will avoid that starving feeling at mealtime thus precluding you from taking in too many calories.

During each meal, you may have the beverage of your choice listed in rule six of the previous chapter.

Eating out. Dining out can be difficult, as restaurants have not yet caught on to cooking in a light fashion. Foods are usually prepared utilizing fattening techniques, with limited choices. Because of this, you should try to make every attempt to restrict your dining in restaurants. That being said, we all eat out at times, especially on vacations and with friends.

When dining out for breakfast, you need to avoid the temptation of having one of those big breakfast combinations you see in many chain restaurants and diners. It was meals like these that got you into this mess. Try to stick to one of the above choices like an eggbeater omelet with some wheat toast. Keep the home fries off the plate.

Fortunately, lunch is somewhat easier as most places now offer at least something you can choose to accomplish your goal. All fast food places now have salads either plain or with grilled chicken. Many corner stores now sell wraps and fruit. Italian restaurants have grilled shrimp or chicken platters in addition to salads and wraps.

Dinner is a bit more challenging. Many people follow the pattern of eating bread, an appetizer, then the main course, followed with the dessert. This is much more then we need, and will throw off your progress. If you are dining with people compassionate to your cause, once seated, immediately tell the waiter not to bring bread, butter or oil to the table. I am sure many of you have the will power to hold out, but just the sight or smell of it will start your gastric juices and bring on hunger. At the same time you are telling the waiter no bread, ask him to bring you a large glass of water and a side salad with a low calorie low fat dressing. This will put something in your stomach to decrease the hunger mechanism while you are waiting for your meal. Remember, a low fat meat or fish for the entree, a vegetable, and tell the waiter not to put the starch on the plate. Do not order appetizers or desserts. Following these dining instructions will help to limit your temptation and keep you out of trouble.

When preparing your meals at home, I can't stress the importance of learning to prepare your meats and vegetables in a nonfattening way. Using marinades, seasonings and other healthy techniques are crucial for your new commitment to your health. If you are going to take this new lifestyle seriously, you will need to enjoy the food you are consuming and to do that takes creativity. Learn how to cook in a healthy fashion and embrace your new healthy life.

No time to cook. There are times where you will be working late or out all day with no time or desire to cook dinner. For these days buy yourself some healthy light frozen dinners and keep them in your freezer. Examples of these would be Lean Cuisine or Weight Watcher Smart One meals. Remember, until you reach your desired weight, you must buy the ones without potatoes or rice. They do exist. You can add a salad with this if you desire. Having these dinners in your freezer will keep you from ordering that chicken parmesan sandwich from the Italian restaurant.

Ordering out. If you do order from a restaurant, keep it light. Grilled shrimp, grilled vegetables, wraps, or a salad, either plain or with grilled chicken, shrimp, tuna, crabmeat, etc.

If you order from a Chinese take out restaurant it must be steamed chicken or shrimp with vegetables, since most foods are cooked in oil.

I think you get the gist of how to eat. Unfortunately, learning what to eat is only a part of the big picture in losing the weight and keeping it off. This is why so many of us gain it back after some partial success.

Now that you have your inspiration, goal, and initial game plan, get started now. As you continue to read, you will learn what else will be needed to complete your journey successfully.

CHAPTER 8

▼

ROADMAP; TESTING, MEDICATIONS, AND HERBAL THERAPY

Often in my practice, I have patients who come to me stating they have been on numerous diets compliantly, and yet can't lose the weight. When I review what they have done usually it is due to following the diet incorrectly, however there are times it is true. When true, I dig deeper often to find medical reasons that the person didn't realize existed. It is for this reason before starting any diet you should see your doctor. During that visit, explain to them that you are starting a new lifestyle of eating in a manner to promote weight loss and will be exercising regularly. Ask them to do lab work that may be related to your obesity, and make sure they feel that it is safe for you to carry out a daily exercise regiment along with your diet.

Most physicians don't practice weight loss management on a regular basis. Many in fact, are obese themselves. It is for this reason that some will not know to order some of the tests I am about to discuss. These tests are often directly or sometimes indirectly related to your obesity, as you will see when you read on.

Tests

The hormone most people know about is related to the **Thyroid gland.** Simply put, this gland controls your metabolism and therefore the speed of your body. Hypothyroidism (under active thyroid gland), is a common disorder that affects up to ten percent of females over the age of fifty. The most prevalent symptom of this disorder is weight gain. You may also get tiredness, thinning of hair, constipation and dry skin to name the most common symptoms. Some people have no specific symptoms and it is discovered in their lab work when checked. There is a thyroid profile that most labs do to check for this disorder but the most sensitive test is called a Thyroid Stimulating Hormone or **TSH** for short. An elevated level of this would mean your thyroid is under active. It is corrected with a simple thyroid supplement that your doctor can prescribe.

Doing this would revert your body's metabolism back to normal.

Lack of **Growth Hormone** can be another etiology for your obesity. Yes even as an adult you have this hormone. Obviously when you are in your childhood, this hormone is very prevalent as you are in your growing years. When we reach adulthood the levels decrease, however there is always a constant amount that is being made. When this level becomes too low, fat content in the body increases, osteoporosis develops, and there is thinning and wrinkling of the skin. Since this hormone is made primarily in your sleep, I find my patients who don't sleep well often have a deficiency in this hormone. When I notice this in my obese patients and further investigate, I discover they often have obstructive sleep apnea. If you have a disruptive sleep, you should make your doctor aware and see if a sleep study should be done on you. The easiest test to check your growth hormone is called **IGF1.** If deficient, your physician may wish to order further testing. This is because there is also something known as hypothalamic obesity. This is very rare but is caused by damage to the part of the brain known as the hypothalamus. Symptoms related may be headaches, blurry vision, vomiting, seizures and somnolence to name a few. If you are truly growth hormone deficient, your doctor may consider ordering further tests and giving you a prescription for this hormone. Growth hormone is given as a subcutaneous injection that you can give to yourself on a daily basis. If you are truly deficient in this hormone and do this, the weight will shed off very easily decreasing fat and increasing muscle mass in your body. In addition, it will reverse osteoporosis and decrease wrinkles. There are people who try to use this for the wrong reasons. I strongly state that you do not do this, as anyone who does not have a true deficiency and uses this can have an increase risk of side effects in the body. The other problem is its extremely high cost and the lack of support with the insurance companies in coverage to pay for this drug. There are people who when tested have levels in the low normal range. In other words just barely making the norm. In these people I advise them to go to their local health food store and buy arginine, ornithine, and lysine. These amino acids along with DHEA and exercise have some suggested evidence of naturally boosting your body's own growth hormone levels. However if your levels are well within the normal range, there is no reason to go out and spend money on something you do not need.

Cortisol has captured the public's eye lately with a barrage of treatments designed to block this product in your body and help you lose weight. Cushing syndrome is a disease characterized by central obesity, hypertension, a plethoric face and atrophy of the skin.

This is a result of pathologically high cortisol levels in your body. When suspected your doctor can do the appropriate testing to evaluate for this syndrome. It is felt however that you don't always need pathologic levels in your body to promote obesity. High normal levels induced by our daily stressful lives of work, bills, problems etc, may be a contributing factor causing increased fat, resistant to dieting. This is why a screening level of this hormone is not unreasonable, especially if hypertension is present. If your level is not pathologic but in the high normal range, you may consider one of these herbal products sold in health food stores that may help block cortisol naturally. As always this should be done under the supervision of your doctor.

Any menopausal female reading this book knows what happens to them when **estrogen** levels drop during this time. Without going into medical details, there is a change in fat distribution and an increase in abdominal fat occurs. Because of possible links to malignancies, taking estrogen has been a hot topic of discussion over the past few years. Recent discussions on this topic blame the synthetic forms of female hormones used in the past. New claims are stating that the use of bioidentical estrogens and progesterone may not carry these risks, however long term studies still need to be concluded. Woman who do use these bioidentical hormones do note reduction in the fat of their abdomen, hips and legs. For a woman who is post-menopausal, foods such as broccoli, apples, celery, yams, cauliflower, cucumbers, squash, cherries, olives, pears, tomatoes plums and especially soy may have a natural estrogen effect on the body and is fine.

What most people don't realize is excess estrogen is becoming a common phenomenon. As Americans, we are consuming environmental estrogens. Much of the turkey and cattle we eat are pumped with estrogen. Doing this makes the animal heavier and tender. In addition, there are also estrogen like compounds in many of the plastics used as containers to store foods. This can become a problem in males and in childhood bearing females. Along with obesity, excess estrogen has been shown to cause low sperm counts and breast development in men. In women, it is linked to pre-menstrual syndrome, and early puberty in young girls.

In my office I have seen cases of obesity linked to high estrogen levels in the body. A simple **estradiol** level can be used. When this is elevated, adjustment of foods to those purely organic must be practiced. In addition, avoidance of storage and heating of foods in plastic containers is necessary. By following this regiment usually over time it is effective. A drug by the name of Arimedex blocks estrogen in your body. Based on your individual medical situation, the use of this drug can be decided by your doctor.

Serotonin is a chemical in your body that makes you feel good when levels are proper. This chemical activates the sympathetic nervous system, which then decreases the feeding mechanism in our body. It also increases our body energy expenditure of calories, making it easier to burn them. When levels of this are off, the opposite can occur. This also can be checked with a simple blood test. Medication such as sibutramine otherwise known as the brand name Meridia will increase serotonin availability to the brain. By doing this it will help decrease your appetite. It will also increase your energy expenditure thereby assisting you in your weight loss. This is a prescription drug that can only be prescribed by your doctor.

Liver function tests are usually part of most screening blood work. It is important that this organ be healthy as one of its many jobs is to help create hormonal balance in your body. When the liver is damaged from alcohol, drugs, chemicals or viruses, its role will be compromised.

Testosterone is another hormone that is important in the obesity arena. Although most people would think that this only would affect men, small amounts are supposed to be present in females. In addition to the commonly known decrease in libido and sexual dysfunction, low levels are associated with decrease in vitality, muscle strength, decline in well being, depressed mood and obesity. A **total testosterone as well as free testosterone** should be checked in the blood. If low, testosterone may be prescribed by your doctor. In men it is crucial to be certain that there is no evidence of prostate cancer prior to its use, as it will act as a fuel for this malignancy. If the prostate is healthy and your levels are truly deficient, this drug can be used with reasonable safety. Currently, there are gel forms of testosterone that are absorbed through the skin designed for males. Unfortunately, there are no such products on the market yet for females. In the meantime if your doctor feels it is medically necessary, a compounding pharmacist can make a special reduced strength designed for women. DHEA, which is a natural precursor to testosterone in the body, can also be purchased at the local health food store. Once again, the importance of discussing this with your doctor must be emphasized.

Metabolic testing is a nice way to evaluate how effective your metabolism is in general. Many people complain of a slow metabolism, but can this be verified? Every person has unique caloric needs. One person may keep their weight stable eating 1800–2200 calories. Another person might be between 2100–2500 calories. Every individual is different. A test called **indirect calorimetry** helps to determine your metabolic rate and your caloric needs for keeping your weight stable as well as what it will take to lose. This machine measures your oxygen consumption and by doing this, can determine resting metabolic rate. Once you have determined this, it can calculate how many calories you need to keep your weight stable and how many you should be consuming to lose. From there it can estimate how many calories you burn with exercise and activities. It can also give a chart of where you compare to another person of typical sex, age, height and weight. Unless you go to a doctor who practices weight loss, chances are he does not have this machine.

Doing this test is helpful not only in your education, but also in helping the physician determine if you truly are one of those people with an abnormally slow metabolism. These are the people who no matter what they do right just can't seem to lose the weight. Usually, they need one of those diet medications for a short time that will help increase their metabolism. This will jump start your body until your metabolic rate can be increased on its own with diet and exercise.

Genes are the new hot topic in the field of obesity. In the past everyone blamed their obesity on their metabolism, now it's their genes. The real story is that there are rare genetic syndromes associated with obesity. All are associated with diminished development of the gonads and display themselves in childhood. There is research in adults that suggests the possibility of genetic mutations that may be present that trigger eating, and decrease energy expenditure and metabolic rate. Without getting into a science lesson here is how I break this all down.

1) If the majority of obesity is genetic, why has it only manifested itself over the past twenty to thirty years? If it were true this would be passed on from generation to generation instead of this recent marked rapid rise.

2) This is a possibility for a small number of the obese people out there.

3) This field of study is still in its childhood stage. As these genes are identified, it will take several years to create, test, and bring to market drugs or methods to counter them. Unfortunately from a genetic standpoint there is nothing you can do.

4) What you can do is realize that it is all the more reason to change your lifestyle. If you are truly genetically programmed to be obese, by eating incorrectly and not exercising you will bring morbid obesity upon yourself and shorten your lifespan. Take the bull by the horns and get yourself to the healthiest weight and best shape your body will permit.

Prescription medication to lose weight is something I am frequently asked about in my medical practice. The reality is only a small percentage of people really need a prescription for this purpose. When done correctly, weight loss is not as difficult as many would think. Unfortunately, people often look for the easy way by turning toward technology to accomplish their goals. Technology is a wonderful thing when used correctly, but should only be used in people who truly need it. As I mentioned a short while ago, **sibutramine** otherwise known under its brand name of **Meridia** in the United States and **Reductil** in Europe is approved for weight loss. This drug is a selective reuptake inhibitor of norepinephine, serotonin, and dopamine. What that means is it works on chemicals in your body to make you want to eat less, and increase your body's energy expenditure so you can burn calories more effectively. As I stated earlier, it is an effective drug when used in the appropriate patient. It does have the potential to raise your blood pressure and heart rate. Therefore, it should be used with caution under physician guidance in people with hypertension. Another down side are the insurance companies once again not wanting to cover it on their formularies. So be prepared to pay for this drug as often times even patients with prescription plans must pay cash. **Orlistat** otherwise known as brand name **Xenical,** and most recently introduced over the counter as **Alli,** is another drug approved for weight loss. This drug decreases the amount of dietary fat that is absorbed in the body by the gastrointestinal tract when you eat. Doing this promotes weight loss, as well as decreasing your lipids, glucose and insulin levels. Side effects are possible loose oily stools, as this is where the fat goes when it is not absorbed. The drug does work but my personal feeling is lets not use technology to decrease the amount of fat absorbed, lets just decrease the amount of fat we eat. Be natural instead of relying on a pill. **Serotonin released anorexants** increase the availability of serotonin in the whole body. Doing this they act as a stimulant and increase the body's metabolism. There are a few of these on the market. One of these dexfenfluramine, was removed from the market for possible complications of valvular abnormalities and pulmonary hypertension. The others on the market have not been proven to cause this, but should be used with caution. These drugs are effective in people who truly have a slow metabolic rate and in my opinion should not be used in any other setting. When used, it should only be for short periods under the observation of your doctor.

Herbal preparations are the next new fad as drug store shelves are full of all kinds of products designed to help people lose weight. These natural products can be of some benefit when used safely with the proper lifestyle of eating correctly and exercise. Unfortunately most people use these as their diet, continue to eat incorrectly and only have partial success. So many commercials on the radio and television with the message to just take these pills and lose the weight has convinced the public that they don't have to eat correctly, just take pills. The problem with these supplements is that they are not regulated by the food and drug administration so their efficacy and safety are a big question mark. This is why it is very important to choose only supplements that you have researched and discussed with your doctor. Doing this you will become educated in knowing all benefits and risks of that product. It is also important to use reputable brands that use reliable manufacturers to make their products.

In this section I am not going to use specific brand names, I will go into the ingredients many of the products use. In the past the most widely used herbal supplements contained ephedra and herbal forms of **caffeine** called guarana and gotu kola. The use of these is derived from ancient Chinese recipes that include an herb called ma huang. Supplements that contain these have been used successfully in the world. Side effects have included dry mouth, insomnia, headaches, hypertension seizures, tachycardia and death. Ephedrine has since been banned in the United States as a supplement to promote weight loss. Many preparations just use regular caffeine as their primary ingredient. Anyone who has used it to stay up all night knows that it increases the body's metabolic rate. It has also been shown to break down fats. Caffeine when used with other herbal products may have a role in assisting a person to lose weight, however they should not be relied upon as the primary tool nor should be used in excess or for long term use. **Green tea extract** is an herb that naturally occurs with caffeine to increase the body's energy expenditure. In my practice I don't advocate finding these herbs on the shelf in pill form, but I tell my patients to enjoy some of the many green teas available on the market with one or two of their meals. As long as they are used in this limited fashion, they can do very little harm and may actually help to some degree. **Hydrosycitric acid** is another product with mixed results found on the shelves. **Capsaicin** derived from the chili pepper may have some effects on increasing the body's metabolism. **Capsinoids** are a family of compounds that are analogs of capsaicin. I would like to see more data before I recommend these, but if you like chili peppers enjoy. Another product known as **5 Hydroxytryptophan or 5 HTP** for short is often found in health food stores. The claim here is taking this will decrease carbohydrate cravings and appetite. Anecdotally, I find some truth to this but a noted side effect is tiredness. I have used this product for patients taking the serotonin released anorexants. It appears to help decrease the jittery feeling sometimes seen with this class of medication. I have made mention earlier about the use of **Arginine, Ornithine, and Lysine** to help stimulate the body's natural growth hormone in people deficient. **Chromium Picolinate** may have some usefulness in stabilizing blood sugars, and decreasing body fat. A noted side effect may be anemia. **DHEA** is a natural occurring hormone in the body, where it is the precursor to testosterone and estrogen. There are many claims to this pill from weight loss to increased libido to helping prevent cancer and heart disease. The verdict in my eyes is still out there on these issues. In my own practice, when I see a patient with a low testosterone level, I will advise using this for a short trial. Anecdotally I find it to have some benefit in this circumstance. **Cortisol blocking products** are hot on the shelves these days using various herbal recipes designed to decrease stress, help manage weight, and boost the immune system. Once again I try to tailor these types of products for the right person. In my practice if a patient already has a reasonable cortisol level there is no point in using something that claims to block it. In the occasional person who fits the right criteria, it can be tried with observation. **Chitsan**

supplements contain fiber from shellfish with the claim of blocking fat absorption, decreasing cholesterol, and promoting weight loss. Side effects may include gas, bloating, and diarrhea. **St. Johns Wort** is another product with claims of decrease appetite and weight loss. I have not seen any study to convince me. **Hoodia** is another product that has not demonstrated to me any significant help with weight loss. There are all kinds of **Bars and Shakes** on the market designed to help you lose weight. Many of these are basically controlled meals, and anytime you practice this technique you will lose weight. The problem with these is you never learn how to eat properly. So after a while you start getting sick of them, and go right back to old incorrect eating habits only to gain back the weight.

As you can see there are a great deal of products on the market each using various formulations claiming to assist in weight loss. The products above are some of the more common ones. There are others, however I didn't want to go on forever on this topic. As obesity increases, sales of these products will follow. The attraction to these products will continue since they are perceived by the public as all natural and assumed to be safer. Some of these formulations appear to increase the body's metabolism. Some claim to help redirect nutrients from fat to muscle, while others claim to help with decreasing appetite by satisfying the stomach. Unfortunately unlike prescription drugs, they are not monitored by the Food and Drug Administration therefore many of the claims have not gone through the scrutiny they deserve before being ingested by the public. When used they should be temporary, under the supervision of your physician, along with learning how to eat correctly and exercise.

CHAPTER 9

ROADMAP; EXERCISE
AND ACTIVITY

In order to lose the weight and change your lifestyle, exercise and increase in activity are vital components in the formula for success. These are two separate individual things, but many people like to think of them as one. Often in my office when I tell patients to exercise, their response is they walk around a lot at work or exercise cleaning the house. These are what I call activities and they are important because they do burn calories. In order to lose the weight quickly and effectively you need to also add exercise. Remember earlier in the book I explained by eating 350 calories less per day would mean it would take you ten days to lose one pound. Adding exercise and activity to your daily regiment can help you change that to a pound every two to three days. In addition to burning calories, exercise will improve your body's metabolism, increase muscle mass, and decrease insulin resistance in your muscles, thereby lowering your blood sugar. It will decrease your cholesterol and improve your cardiopulmonary health. Doing this will help you breathe better and decrease your risk for heart attack and stroke. It will also improve your overall well being, because people who exercise just feel better and have more energy.

So how much exercise should be done and what kind should it be? First and foremost I need to repeat, let your doctor know what you intend to do so he may help guide you. This is to make sure medical conditions don't preclude you from doing certain things. For example, if you have debilitating arthritis you may not be able to do certain exercises that will increase stress on the affected joints. A program of physical therapy prescribed by your doctor may be helpful in improving this and make it easier to do other things. In addition, if during exercise you experience chest discomfort, unusual shortness of breath or pain anywhere, inform your doctor immediately so that appropriate testing and treatment may be undertaken.

The next thing you need to assess is where you are at the current moment. Are you someone who can walk for thirty minutes straight without stopping? You may be someone who can do only ten minutes at a time. For people who are very limited at first, I find that starting off a little at a time is appropriate. This is not a race, this is something that hopefully you will have a very long life doing. For my patients with limitations, I will usually tell them to start with ten minutes a day of something (details to come in a little bit). Do this for one week, after which slowly try to stretch it a little longer than the ten minutes by doing it twice a day. By week three you should be at fifteen minutes twice a day. Eventually as time goes by you will be able to do the thirty minutes in one clip. Excuses for not doing exercise are common as I hear all of them in my office:

1) I work too much

2) My kids keep me to busy to exercise

3) I don't have money to join a gym or buy equipment

4) It's too hot or too cold outside to walk

5) Etc etc etc

My response to these people is I work at least 54 hours a week from Monday though Friday along with another 10 to 12 hours every other weekend. In between I take calls from patients and families and I have 2 children who have been active in sports that I do not miss. I have a wife who I value and try to spend time going out with and I am writing this book. Through all this, I exercise for 30 to 45 minutes 4 times a week faithfully. It is a must in my schedule. The only way I can do all of these activities is because of exercise. It gives me the energy to take care of myself so I can be vibrant and alert throughout each day. During any times where I have slipped from my exercise regiment for a little bit, I found myself tired, lazy and irritable. I am sure many of you have experienced these emotions, which when left to continue, often lead to a feeling of depression. Lets break though some of these barriers.

1) I work too many hours

As I mentioned so do I, but lets look at what most people do. They wake up in the morning at 6:30 or so to get ready for work that starts at 8:00. Unfortunately, many of us have longer work hours or commute, which prevents us from coming home until 7:00 at night. We order take out or cook something quick that is usually fattening. From there we talk to our children or go on the phone with friends, or maybe straighten up the house for a little bit. From 8:00 until 11:00 at night we watch one television show after another, as this is our "downtime to relax". It's down time all right because it is bringing you right down the drain. It is time to make some changes in your life.

Unless you are one of those people that start work at 5:00 AM, I find that waking up 35 minutes earlier and exercising in the morning is best. Although hard at first, it will give you energy for the daytime and give you that nice healthy tired feeling at night so you can sleep better. So instead of getting up at 6:30, wake up at 5:55 AM. Stretch your muscles for 5 minutes and then exercise for the next 30 minutes each day. You will follow your new dietary habits for the day. After dinner, consider increasing your activities by doing something with your family. After a few days, you will find yourself tired and going to bed about thirty minutes earlier as your body will soon adjust to the time change. You will also notice you will sleep better at night.

2) My kids keep me too busy to exercise

For those of you with kids who cannot follow the above regiment, once again there are no excuses. People always assume that exercise has to be something structured, like going to a gym or walking on a treadmill. Those who make that assumption are wrong. In fact, exercise often times can be incorporated with your children. As they see what you do, maybe they too will adapt this good habit. If your children are infant age, putting them in a carriage and taking a fast walk will satisfy this purpose. As they get older you can play with them. Go in the back yard and play tag or other games. Take them to a pool and swim with them. Turn swimming into a game by racing them back and forth. If you want to really exercise, teach them how to ride a bike. As you run along side of them, you will get a good work out. Once they know how to ride, go riding with them. If they like a particular sport teach them and work with them. Doing these things, will teach them to move their bodies and keep themselves physically fit. When they get older, if they are playing organized sports like my children did, use this time effectively. When you bring them to their practices, instead of sitting on the side talking with the other parents gossiping or complaining about the coach, go for a power walk. On game days it is usually mandatory to get there thirty to forty minutes early. Use this time for your walk so when the game starts you are right there watching. This was my regular routine in all the years both my children were active. As I would do this I would watch all the overweight parents standing around chatting, eating, and smoking.

3) I don't have money to join a gym or buy equipment

People today are so caught up in joining a gym or buying fancy machines at lofty prices. This is a nice luxury, but not a necessity as you can see from the examples of exercise mentioned. If you feel you need a structured program with trainers and machines and fortunate enough to afford it, by all means indulge yourself. They can sometimes be helpful in improving muscular tone. If your goal is simply to get in shape and be healthy, anything that gets your heart rate up for 30 to 45 minutes will do the job just fine. I personally do not have a membership to a gym. I do own an elliptical machine, a stationary bike and some weights that I sometimes use. I prefer doing a combination of walking and running, especially with my dogs. Since I work primarily indoors, I love to bike, or go hiking because it gives me the opportunity to enjoy some fresh air and the great outdoors.

4) It's too hot, It's too cold

Living in the northeast, the months of July, August, January February can be extreme. There are still no excuses. Early mornings and evenings in the summer tend to be more tolerable. In the winter you can exercise in the house. There are all kinds of exercise programs that you can buy on DVD that are inexpensive allowing you to follow a formalized workout program right in front of your television. If you do have the money to buy a machine of some sort, buy one. If it is close to your birthday or the upcoming holidays tell your family to buy you one.

5)Etc, etc, etc

As you can see, where there is a will there is a way. You have to stop making one excuse after another. In life there are those who do, and those who make excuses. Be the former and get healthy.

What kind of Exercise?

Each person is different depending on age, the extent of your obesity, and underlying medical problems. If you do have significant medical problems your doctor can be of some help in this area. If you have no restrictions and are at an age where you are still active, I find team sports are a great way to force you to stick to a schedule. Joining a basketball or flag football league where people are dependant on you to show up provides that often needed incentive. If this is not an option, as I stated earlier biking, hiking and power walking are wonderful forms of exercise that get you fresh air. If you are willing to spend the money for something in the house, my personal preference is to purchase an elliptical machine. These are the machines with the handgrips and foot pedals that go simultaneously. The advantage of these machines is you are using and toning the muscles of both upper and lower body. This is in contrast to walking or biking where you are primarily using only the lower section of your body. This machine also has little impact on your hips, back, knees and ankles. For many obese people this is an important factor as years of being overweight has caused grinding and damage to these joints causing pain and discomfort when walking. Stomp your foot once on the ground and you can feel the vibration on the knee. This impact when done on a person of normal weight is minimal, but in the obese can often cause pain. Other forms of low impact exercises are biking, swimming and steppers.

Good old fashion walking is a wonderful way to get started for most people. Although there is some impact, it is tolerable to most people providing a cheap quick way to get started on your new lifestyle journey. It should be done at a brisk pace. It is not a stroll in the mall. In addition, to help tone your upper body, bring those little mini three pound weights with you. Put one in each hand and swing your arms in a curling type motion while doing your daily walk.

How much?

When people think about exercise they usually associate a frequency of 3 to 4 times a week as the proper amount. This number is correct if you are talking about improving your cardiovascular and pulmonary conditioning. It is a good number when you wish to stay in shape and this is how often I exercise. However, there is a difference between this and losing weight. Remember you have gone far off the road and to get back on you have some catching up to do. If you want to lose weight you have to exercise every day. You read correctly, everyday. I understand a day once a week may slip by due to some event going on in your life, but a daily regiment should be your goal.

As I stated earlier, many who are obese are not physically fit, so it will take time to build up to where you need to be. Start off with 20 minutes per day. You may divide this into 2 sessions if doing this in one is too much. As this becomes a ritual, you will begin to notice the weight and inches coming off nicely, as you firm up those flabby areas of your body. All exercise should be done at a moderate pace. As I said before it is not a stroll in the mall, however you don't have to kill yourself either. People who try to over do it often times injure themselves by straining or pulling muscles. Doing this will make you unable to continue and ruin your progress. So remember, moderation is the key to life. Losing weight often comes in spurts with periods of drops and then a sudden stall. This is your body bucking you, telling you have been this way for a long time, are you sure you want to change. You will notice in the first couple of weeks the weight will come off easy. This will occur as you slowly increase your exercise. After a month or so the weight loss may start to slow down. This is a sign that your body is beginning to resist, and it is usually the point where you are tolerating the 20 minutes a day. It is time for you to increase your exercise to 30 minutes a day to get back on track. This is necessary because the increase in exercise will not only burn more calories, but will increase your body's metabolic rate helping you to burn calories easier. For most people the 30 minutes may be adequate for a lifetime. In some who have a tremendous amount to lose, a few months go by and then you sometimes hit another brick wall of not losing weight. It will be time to kick it up a notch once again. Hopefully by now, you will be enjoying the exercise, and it should not be a chore anymore. As it becomes part of your routine, it should be making you feel better as it gives you vigor in your daily activities. It will be at this time, that you will need to increase it to 45 minutes a day. By now your muscles are starting to show themselves. As you are losing inches and fat, you are gaining muscle, which may increase your weight. If the area of your upper arms called the biceps and triceps use to be fat, and with exercise has become muscle, this area weighs more the when you started. This is a good thing, as all these areas of flabby fat are converted to lean muscle. What use to be jiggling when you moved, will now be nice and firm. When you exercise, not only will your outer muscles get stronger and more efficient, but your heart and lungs will also. Exercise makes your heart's muscle becomes stronger, allowing it to pump blood easier. Once this happens it can work less by doing the same job with less beats. This is why someone who is athletic has a slow pulse rate. It can now do the same job in sixty beats that an out of shape heart will do in eighty beats or more. As this occurs your blood pressure starts to decrease and so does your risk of heart attack and stroke. Your muscles will use the sugar in your blood for these activities and decrease their resistance to insulin, thereby making your blood glucose levels decrease. Any diabetic reading this book can reproduce this by simply taking your blood sugar with a finger stick. After doing so, exercise for 30 minutes then retake your glucose level. The drop in the number will astound you. Do this regularly and watch the numbers go down even more. So remember when you hit this second wall, tell your body that you are going to break through it and continue on the path of losing weight and better health. This is not a diet, this is a change of lifestyle where exercise will be a permanent part of the new you. This is a time in your life where you are losing weight, inches, getting firmer, and ridding your arteries of all the fat build up. It is the new you.

As I mentioned earlier, in my office when I ask people it they are exercising, they respond by saying they walk around a lot at work. This is not exercise because it does not accomplish the goals above that require you to get your heart rate up for 30 to 45 minutes continuously on a regular basis. This does count as an increase in activity.

Activity plays a vital role in the weight loss process. If you recall earlier, I mentioned that an additional 400–700 calories each day potentially burn as you increase your body motion. People who have jobs that require them to move around have a tremendous advantage to people who sit at a computer all day. Look at the people who have heavy labor jobs and you will note that most are not obese. The ones who are overweight eat horribly. Unfortunately, most of our manufacturing has left the country and the ones that have stayed are usually automated assembly. This is why it becomes our job to make sure we increase our body motion. When feasible and safe, use the stairs instead of the elevator. The same pertains to finding a parking space a little further away. Start cleaning the closets and windows in your home. Do some backyard work. Get out of the car instead of using the drive though window. Get the idea. With each body movement, calories will be used to accomplish it. Every time it adds up to 3500, another pound is gone. It really is that simple and further conveys the point; it's not just what you eat but also what you burn. While in medical school, my sister once asked one of her teaching physicians how he stays so energetic and in shape. His response is one I would I would like to share. "When I feel like lying down I sit. When I feel like sitting I stand. When I feel like standing I walk. When I feel like walking I jog and when I feel like jogging I run." Learn to develop the habit of increasing your body's movement and activity, and watch as you transform yourself to health.

Focus point # 8) Write down how you will accomplish your exercise goals. List ways you will be able to increase your body's activities. Look at these regularly and stick to it faithfully.

CHAPTER 10

▼

BELIEF

There are millions of people who believe they are overweight due to factors they have no control over. "It's my genes. My parents never taught me how to eat. I can't change because this is who I am. Food gives me comfort." One negative belief after another rules their minds converting them into the person that they are. Say it a few more times and you'll believe it, is an old saying that people say in jest that has validity. Our mind will take whatever constructive or destructive thoughts we feed it and turn it into reality. Why does the thought of skydiving from a plane bring different emotions from different people? Some have fear, and yet others pure exhilaration. It is all in the belief of what skydiving is to that person. If you feel skydiving will be exhilarating, it will be. If you are fearful, it will never happen. The same is true of weight loss. If you hang on to negative beliefs, you will have a poor outcome. If you believe that you have the ability to make the changes necessary for success, you will find your pot of gold. Furthermore, if you believe it will change your life for the better and losing the weight can be an enjoyable process, it will be. In life, success and failure are the products of your thoughts.

Often times our faith is hindered by fears. Fear that we can't accomplish the overall task and ultimate failure. What you need to know is everyone fails at times. You will make mistakes on this journey called weight loss. If you truly believe that you can get back on track and do so, success will follow.

Another belief people frequently have is that food brings them comfort. Many people eat when they are stressed, upset, angry, nervous, or have feelings of inadequacy. They feel that eating relieves this negative in their life and brings them pleasure. The food is their comfort and therapy. Having this association has taken you down the wrong road. It may have given you some temporary solace, but ultimately it has taken you to a place you don't want to be. It is time to create some new beliefs for these situations. It is time to believe when you are stressed, that eating takes you to a worse place of depression, low self-esteem, and poor health.

From now on, when you feel these things you will exercise, meditate, do yoga, or anything that has a positive effect on the body. You can choose from any number of things as long as it doesn't make your health get worse. It is time to start to analyze some of the negative beliefs you may have and create new positive ones.

Focus point # 9) Write down all of the negative beliefs you have had about yourself in the past and what they have cost you.

You know what these are. I can't lose weight because _____belief

Train yourself to have new beliefs and the new things they will bring you. Understand that you value food, but your most important belief is in your health. Then use your new food style to support your beliefs. Believe that when you eat correctly it will change your life for the better. Believing that the journey can be done is crucial to your success. Once you have your beliefs written, reaffirm and say them to yourself on a daily basis. Repetition of your new beliefs into your mind is a crucial process in ridding those old negative ones that have lingered there for so long.

Focus point #10) Write down a new set of positive beliefs and what they will bring you. Remember to reaffirm them daily.

Whatever you want in life requires a necessary action. Something as simple as wanting a quart of milk requires some time and effort to get in your car or walk to the store to get it. If you want to be a movie star, you have to make changes and take action to begin whatever steps are necessary to achieve that goal. <u>So what do you want?</u> Do you want to be thin and healthy? If this is what you want, bite the bullet and start taking the steps needed to achieve your goal. **Decide what you want, then do what is necessary to make it work.**

CHAPTER 11

▼

MISTAKES, WRONG TURNS AND BUMPS IN THE ROAD

You now have the basic knowledge it takes to lose weight. If you follow the rules and regulations and stay on the course of your new lifestyle change, not only will the weight come off, you will become a new person.

The problems you will face will be going off course, making wrong turns and having blips where the weight may not be coming off. Sometimes it is by mistake, as you may eat something incorrectly without realizing it was not conducive to weight loss. Many times it is the little devil on your left shoulder convincing you that it is ok to eat the wrong foods. He whispers in your left ear how good you've been all week. He asks why you are depriving yourself. It's just one ice cream cone or one piece of cake goes through your mind as you are convinced you are not doing any harm, and will make up for it tomorrow. Other times you are doing everything right. You are just not having the success you should have, or all of a sudden something happened and the weight loss stops. These are the bumps in the road and wrong turns on the trip to Boston. When these things happen, you can give up, turn around and go home, or you can see where you veered off course, learn from your mistake, and get back on the correct road to complete your journey. Sadly, too many times most people say oh well, I messed up, and go back to their old bad ways of eating. The other common mistake comes when you are doing well. It starts one day with one little thing that you know is wrong. Soon after, you continue to sabotage yourself, dabbling with incorrect food that soon brings you back to your old ways. Within a couple of weeks the weight loss stops. By the third week, you are not weighing yourself anymore because you are gaining and no one likes to see failure. In my office the people who fail follow this pattern. During week one of the cheating they come in with their diary because there are only a few mistakes and the weight loss is minimal. On week two they forget their diary and there is no weight loss. On the third week they don't show up for their appointment, only to be seen a couple of months later for a cold or other medical problem. It is at that visit that the weight lost has been gained back and then some, as they are loaded with the typical alibis. Work got busy, family stress, my boss, my kids, sick relative, family reunion, and barbeques, are some of the few. Every once and a while someone will step up, accept the blame and take responsibility for themselves. These are the ones who start again and have success.

Focus point #11) People who are successful with anything in life don't make excuses when things go wrong. They accept the result, analyze what went wrong, fix it and move on. Do the same with your food habits and new life.

Let's go through how to handle the mistakes, wrong turns and bumps in the road.

You ate the wrong things by mistake.

This is the where the value of your diary will show itself. Eating without writing down what you are doing gives you no way to analyze what you were doing wrong if the weight loss stops. Even if you think you remember, it's not to what degree and how often.

Having a diary will give you the ability to visualize everything that you put in your mouth everyday. It will allow you to retrospectively go through your meals. What you thought was an occasional cheat, becomes frequent when you review it on paper. When you look back you will find food that you are uncertain about. Doing this you can review chapter six or the outline at the end of the book to see if the foods in question were permissible. After you review, you can learn from your mistakes with the knowledge of what you did incorrectly. At that point you can pick up from where you left off and get back on the right road to your destination. This process is invaluable as it will allow recall of your meals as well as reinforce your knowledge by constantly reviewing the material.

The Little Devil

This one is a little tougher as your brain is trying to get you off course. Here your mind is trying to sabotage your success. When this occurs it is time to dig deeper to try and learn why you do the things you do.

Once again, the diary can be an important tool to show you when you cheated and how it occurred. Knowing this, you can usually remember what the circumstances were. You will notice it occurred during stressful times at work or when relaxing in front of the television. Maybe it occurs at parties or with friends who are trying to get you to eat like them? Many times it is your own body trying to convince you that you deserve those little pleasures. The diary will track your failures and then it will be up to you to determine what you really want. Do you want pleasure for the short term, or the long term? If it is the short term, don't whine and complain about your weight and be prepared for the consequences. If it is the long term, become aware of the little devil on your shoulder and through your failures train yourself for success. When you review your diary, circle the foods that were the culprits and think about what made you go off course. Realize that it was this line of thinking and these foods that got you to this place you don't like in your life. Train your mind to realize that this bad state you are in of tiredness, huffing and puffing, and possibly taking medication comes from that little devil telling you that you deserve that ice cream.

Typically the little devil comes out around the third week. During the first couple weeks you are usually very inspired and well behaved. By the third week you are longing for some of your old habits of eating as you have had some success but not yet felt the full positive effects of your new lifestyle. If you catch yourself in advance, think about what I have just said. If you already gave in and ate incorrectly for whatever reason, you must learn from the experience and move on. One way to learn is to notice how you felt when you cheated. After eating correctly for a few weeks, eating fatty type foods tends to make you feel bloated and sluggish. Pay attention to this difference, your body is trying to tell you something. Look at your diary and circle the things you did wrong. After you do that, weigh yourself and see what that food does to you. Think about what triggered the action to eat that way. Create ways to avoid these triggers. If it is certain beliefs that are the trigger, try to create new ones. For example, using the belief that when stressed, you have to eat something sweet. Take that belief and attach a negative outcome to it. Change it to when stressed, you eat something sweet, gain weight and then feel bad about yourself. Once that is done attach a new belief. When you feel stressed, you will have a healthy sweet like an apple, and exercise to work off this emotion. This will satisfy your craving and make you look and feel better.

Making these changes won't be easy but they must occur to have success. You can't leave things the same and expect miracles. If you keep things the same, things stay the same. So make some real changes in your beliefs and listen to the angel on the right shoulder and not the devil on the left one. **Remember the little devil of temptation got you to where you are now.**

Not Losing Weight From The Start

You are following the rules and diet plan. You are keeping a diary and analyzing it to make certain the foods you ate were correct. You are exercising regularly and increasing your activity. Doing all this and not losing weight usually indicates that there is something medically wrong. As I mentioned in chapter eight, there are a number of medical conditions that can affect your weight. If you recall, an underactive thyroid gland, lack of growth hormone, serotonin irregularities, elevated cortisol, liver dysfunction, estrogen abnormalities, testosterone deficiency, and a slow metabolism are all possibilities that can play a role in obesity. Often, medications used by physicians have weight gain as a side effect. Often times it is minimal, however they may hinder your ability to lose. Glucocorticoids, which are in the steroid family, dominate this list of drugs. An example of this would be prednisone. Phenothiazines, and other anti-psychotic medications such as Amitriptiline and Nortriptiline also cause weight gain. Blood pressure and heart medications called beta and alpha blockers, have been implicated in this process. Anti epileptic medication, with the exception of topiramate, have been implicated in weight gain. Most diabetic medication with the exception of metformin, has been shown to cause weight gain. Medications that stimulate appetite such as megestrol and cyproheptadine obviously will cause weight gain.

Understand that these medications have been prescribed by your doctor and are probably necessary for you to take. **Never stop any prescribed medication without the consent of your doctor, as this could be dangerous.** It can't hurt to have a discussion with your doctor to see if there is another medication that could be used in its place. In addition, if you are pregnant or have a psychiatric disorder, any particular diet or change in eating habits may be dangerous, and must be done with the consent and close monitoring of your physician.

So if you are not losing from the start, make an appointment to see your physician to discuss your dilemma. Make sure there are no medical reasons for your problem.

Resistance.

This is another one of those things that starts to come into play after following the program for a few weeks. Not only do I hear it a lot in my office, I expect it. "I like the foods I eat. I can't follow this. I don't like that food. I have no time." The list goes on. Basically what you are telling me is you have been following certain habits for so long that you are resistant to change. I realize that change is something that doesn't come easy to anyone. The reason is doing what we have always done is comfortable to us. The way we eat, amongst many things are like an old pair of comfortable slippers. It's time to really look at what these habits have cost us and break through your resistance to change. You have to realize that nothing is free in life so there will be some initial discomfort. If you want to make a change for the better, you have to make a change for the better. It will all be worth it as you see the success. When this happens you will start to enjoy your new lifestyle and be grateful you made the change.

Focus point # 12) If you stray off your diet or develop resistance, you need to brush it off and immediately focus on getting back on track.

Chapter 12

▼

Staying Focused and Persistent

In order to have success that will last, you will need to remain persistent and focused with your new way of thinking. As you move along and thrive in your success, you will constantly have people who will tell you "come on and have a few potato chips." "You already lost all that weight, a few ribs at a party won't change anything". They are wrong, it will change your way of thinking. In your new healthy lifestyle, you have to think like a healthy person. When a person says they are going to diet, it implies a temporary measure to lose some weight. Diets are for people who are already thin, but may have gone on vacation, gained a few pounds and now want to knock it off. If you are consistently overweight, or obese and wish to lose weight and keep it off, do not say you are on a diet. Instead you have to say you are changing your lifestyle. You have decided to live the life of a healthy person, and are dedicated to your new way of living. In order to do this it will require a great amount of focus and persistence to reach your goal.

Unfortunately, failure is the norm when people are trying to change. Failure can come for many reasons.

1) **Lack of Desire.** Most people don't start off in any endeavor hoping to fail. Most lack the desire it takes to be successful. They start off doing what they are supposed to, but when things start to get tough, they cave in. They want to lose the weight, but are not willing to do what is necessary. They talk the talk but don' t want to walk the walk.

2) **Procrastination.** Time and time again in my office when I tell people it is time to lose weight, I hear words along these lines. "I'm going to start right after the holidays." "Right after the summer, right after my vacation, as soon as the kids start school." The list goes on and on. There is no such thing as a bad time to start being a healthy person, just start.

3) **Excuses.** Once again like a broken record in my office, "I was at a party." "Work is too stressful."

"There were too many barbeques this summer". Stop finding the reasons you can't lose and write down why you must change your lifestyle.

4) **Ready to give up.** To many, dieting is just a phase that people go through every so often to comply with the social norm. Unfortunately, because their heart is not in making that commitment to change for the long term, they are ready to chuck it at the first obstacle that presents itself. One party with a lot of fattening food is all it takes to go back to your old ways.

5) **Hoping instead of doing.** So many people tell me that they hope to lose a few pounds, or they are going to try. Look around at successful people, not just in the weight loss genre, but also in life. They don't start their journey hoping or trying to get there. They start with the intent of getting there and do it.

6) **Lack of planning.** This topic is a major concept of this book. Too many people randomly just start a diet without the steps and game plan laid out. Hopefully this book will help prevent this from happening to you.

7) **Looking for the easy way out.** The fad diets and shelves full of diet pills in the drug stores are exhorting money from people who are always look-

ing for the easy way. This is a common feature of many of the baby boomers. Because we are the most educated generation, we are always looking for an easier way of doing things. In many aspects this is a good thing, as it has lead to many of the great advances in technology that we now live with.

When it comes to your body, sometimes simple is just better. There can be no substitution for eating correctly, exercise and activity. It has to be done the old fashion way. Healthy living shouldn't be complicated, so get back to the basics and enjoy the process.

Developing a healthy weight requires not only an understanding as to why you need to change and the knowledge of how to do it, but also a complete transformation in the way you think. It has to be something you enjoy doing, as it becomes fun to watch your waistline drop and have more energy. You begin to love receiving compliments from people as they begin to notice.

So lets change your way of thinking. As I stated earlier, first you have to lose that mindset of you are going to try to change, and transform it to you will change. To do this, you must first learn to remember to link pain to those foods of the past. Link those spareribs, rib eye steaks, cake and ice cream to your obese state, medication, pain and dissatisfaction you feel right now. Whatever went through your mind that brought you to this book, link it to the foods you were enjoying since they are what brought you here. Develop a habit of linking foods like grains, vegetables, fruits, and meats like chicken, turkey and fish to good health, energy and the goals you wish to accomplish. When you have done this you will have achieved a change in your focus. A new way of thinking designed to change the way you perceive things all around you.

Focus point # 13) Link your old habits to your current state of pain and your new habits to your future success.

This is not a diet it is a lifestyle change. Learn to do the opposite of what you did in the past. Remember where that old path took you. When you are tired and feel like you want to sit around, get up and move your body. Go for a walk or do some activity. When you are stressed or angry, instead of sitting around complaining about it on the phone with friends, work it off. You will begin to notice that the exercise will clear your mind and give you more energy to continue on your way to good health. Don't walk around being slow, depressed, sluggish, overweight, and unhappy. Be vibrant, alive and energetic. Stop turning to food for comfort. Always think of the outcome of your actions.

Focus point # 14) Don't focus on your weight, focus on your health and success

When you focus on your weight, it is a constant battle. Most people don't like to fight because it creates displeasure. When this occurs, eventually you will capitulate for the sake of inner peace and return to what was comfortable. If you focus on your obesity and weight, this entire process will be a sacrifice and it is destined for failure. When you focus on your health and well being, you will do the things that you associate to that emotion. I don't think that anyone would argue that eating correctly with exercise and a proper weight are in that line of thought. When you focus on being healthy, you will eat what is in accordance to those thoughts and the success will follow because you will become a product of how you think. Whatever we focus on will occur. Act like you are healthy and the right foods will enter your lifestyle.

Don't be obsessed with the weekly results of the scale. There will be some weeks where a lot will come off, and others where it is a little. It doesn't matter, just stay on course, watch for mistakes and keep chipping away. Eventually you will have success. Ben Franklin once said, "It is true there is much to be done, and perhaps, you are weak handed; but stick to it steadily, and you will see great effects; for constant dropping wears away stones; and by diligence and patience the mouse ate in two the cable; and little strokes fell great oaks."

If you were ever in great shape in your past, and have a photo of this, put it on your refrigerator as a reminder of how you could be if you did the right things. If this is not the case, I want you to think of a movie star or someone who is in great physical shape. Use a picture of them on your refrigerator. Try to think how a person like that might eat. Would it be some fattening bloated meal or something healthy? I always think it is funny when my overweight patients say to me, "You don't have to worry, because you're already thin." The fact of the matter is, I focus my attention on living a healthy lifestyle and being an example to my patients. I eat right, exercise and stay active. By doing these things it keeps my weight in a correct zone. To have success that will last, you have to study and understand this new lifestyle. You can't become a billionaire if you can't think like one. The same holds with your weight and health. Read about health related topics instead of reading about what Britney Spears did this week. Look up new recipes and find cooking books that use healthy ways to prepare meals. Remember, even after you have reached your goal weight and can begin to eat some of the foods denied, you will never be allowed to prepare them in unhealthy fattening ways. Focus on new patterns, where old patterns had you eating. Strive for success to create the new you and enjoy the ride. As you take on this new focus, you will stop thinking what is wrong with you and the better health will soon follow. You will stop focusing on why you are so obese, and change it to look how healthy you are becoming. If you do something incorrectly, analyze what you did and what line of thinking brought you to that line of action. If it was a belief, change it. If it was a habit, change it. Whatever it was, figure it out and create a new line of thought or pattern to correct it so in the future it will not occur. Pay attention, analyze, learn and create new patterns. <u>Leave no doubt in your mind that you can change.</u> Create new patterns of eating that now match your new healthy lifestyle. As I have stated, I have worked with many patients in the process of losing weight. Only the patients that have changed their thoughts and actions were successful for the long term. Focusing on being overweight will make you dwell on the negative and be destined for failure. Without a change in focus only short gains will be achieved. It's time to take control of your life. Don't be a passenger, be the driver of your thoughts and actions. Focus on health and success and you will find it will bring you those things not only with your weight, in all aspects of your life.

While in New Orleans recently, I bought a shirt with the statement "Own Your Life" written across it. This shirt is the essence of what I am trying to tell you in this book. Don't be a victim of the thoughts society has put on you. If there is one thing in this world you should own, it's control of your own life, especially when it comes to your health. So take control and own your life.

Focus point #15) In all aspects in life, remember the steps for success.

CHAPTER 13

▼

YOU'VE REACHED
YOUR GOAL
MAINTENANCE

Congratulations, you've completed your journey and made it to the weight you desire. Preferably, it is one with a BMI of less then twenty-five. By now you should be feeling better. You should have more energy and should be receiving compliments from people, especially from those who have not seen you in a while. If you were on medications in the beginning, hopefully some, if not all, have been removed by your doctor. By now your hips, back and knees should be feeling better with improved mobility. All in all, hopefully you feel like a new person. One who is confident and thinks with a new perspective, focusing on the most important thing in life, your health.

I promised you when you reached your goal, that you would get back some of the foods you had to give up to achieve your mission.

Your new rules and regulations to eating
Rule # 1) Water

Water should always remain a constant in your life. It is healthy and natural and what God created for you to drink. It will continue to serve you as an appetite suppressant, and help with your bowels and kidneys. Continue this good habit you have developed.

Rule # 2) The change in carbohydrates

It is now time to include some of the carbohydrates you had to give up in order to lose weight. I'm not talking about the processed snack foods that will cause immediate weight gain. I am referring to some of those starches that everyone misses so much. This time however, you will learn to eat them without the fat mixed in. In addition, since you are now adjusted to eating more vegetables on your plate, you will naturally limit these starches to smaller portions. Lets start with a potato. It is now ok to have a small portion of potatoes with your dinner. The potato can be baked or boiled with a small amount of margarine or spices if you desire. It can't be cooked in oil or smothered in butter and sour cream. Nor can they be mixed with mayonnaise for potato salad or combined with milk and butter to make them mashed. It is the combining of fat with the starch that will make you start to gain weight again.

A small amount of juice can be added to your diet on occasion, just remember these are concentrated calories and it takes several oranges to make one glass. So in essence you get the calories of several oranges with one serving. If you truly miss juice, you can restart, but keep it to a minimum or consider some of the new light juices recently introduced in the marketplace.

Pasta may now come back into your diet. It is low in fat, however when you eat too much you are what I call "carb loading." When your body consumes too many carbohydrates, it will subsequently convert whatever is not used into fat for storage. So if you really miss your pasta, here is what you do. If you know early in the day that you are going to eat pasta that evening, avoid carbohydrates earlier in the day. Instead of cereal for breakfast and a sandwich at lunch, have eggbeaters, low fat cottage cheese, or a low carb yogurt for breakfast. Then for lunch have a grilled chicken salad or something similar. By dinnertime, you will have eaten very little carbohydrates that day, so they won't be as burdensome to your body. Naturally a grain or wheat pasta will have a better impact on the body than traditional pastas. However, having regular pasta for someone who is not a diabetic is not a terrible thing on occasion. Remember this is not a daily thing. In addition, learn to combine the pasta with some protein and other foods that are not fattening. Let me explain. If you just have a big bowl of pasta, you are consuming one hundred percent carbohydrates for dinner. If you combine this pasta with oil or pork sausage, you are adding too much fat, which is no good. However, if you add some shrimp, chicken or turkey sausage in a light tomato sauce with a salad on the side, you have changed the dynamics of the meal. Instead of having a one hundred percent carbohydrate meal, you are now having a meal consisting of sixty percent carbohydrates, some of which is roughage in the salad, thirty percent protein and ten percent fat. This combination is much more conducive to keeping the body at a neutral weight.

Rice is another starch that many enjoy and may once again be added to your regular diet. Dark rice is preferred, and again care must be used in its preparation.

It is vital to remember when reintroducing these starches into your diet, to cook them in a nonfattening way. The other crucial factor is to practice portion control on the dinner plate.

Processed sugars should never be used anymore because they accelerate weight gain, and are unhealthy. Cereals should continue to be a part of your breakfast life. You can now add those rice and corn cereals you may have been missing. The rule against sweetened kids cereals remains intact.

Continue your use of vegetables and fruit, they are natural and will continue to satisfy you in a healthy way.

Rule #3) Use of Fats

Meats that have large quantities of fats such as processed meats, rib eye steaks, prime rib, most pork dishes need to remain off your diet. The problem with animal fat is it is saturated which is the worst type. If however you find yourself at a party, or a restaurant that specializes in spare ribs, enjoy and focus on the fact that this one time is a treat and will not become a habit. You should also practice some portion control during this time. You will notice since you have been eating well for so long, that eating this type of food will make you feel bloated and sluggish. Pay attention to this, it is your body telling you something. Record it in your mind for future reference.

When it comes to fats in food, you want to look at foods that limit transfats, and are mostly polyunsaturated. Continue to limit frying foods in oils and animal fat. You may begin to use oils that are polyunsaturated or monounsaturated such as safflower, corn, or olive oils for salads and other venues.

For those of you who missed your cheese, here is an opportunity to get something back. There are brands of fat free cheese on the market. These are generally made out of protein. I didn't want you eating them during the weight loss phase for two reasons. First since regular cheese is just a block of fat, I wanted to break the cheese habit for those who love it. I wanted to rid this concept from your taste buds. Early in a diet when you eat traditionally fatty foods converted into a nonfattening design, you are continuing a habit of eating the type of food you enjoyed. When you break your diet, out of habit, you go right back to your old ways of eating the real thing. Secondly, the cheese had additional calories you didn't need when trying to lose the weight. Now that the weight is gone and you have grown accustomed to other foods, use the fat free cheese in limited amounts if you desire.

The same concept is true with real butter. It too is a block of saturated fat. I want you to continue to use margarines. Choose the ones made with polyunsaturated oils.

Rule # 4) Carbs mixed with Fats

This dangerous combination remains on the never eat list. Eating foods like chocolate, ice cream, cookies, cakes, chips, etc should never return to your new lifestyle. If they do, so will the weight.

Rule # 5) Limit Salt

By now you should be adjusted to living life without salt. There is plenty of salt in the foods you eat. Continue to try to avoid.

Rule # 6) Drink Healthy

Gone are the days of soda and sugar drinks. Continue your life of flavored waters, club soda, teas, etc.

Rule # 7) Use Healthy Condiments

Now that you have adjusted to the use of utilizing herbs, spices and marinades that are healthy, you should make every attempt to continue this practice. The one exception may be the limited use of some of the polyunsaturated or monounsaturated oils. I am not talking about going back to frying foods in oil, or dousing your salad in it. I'm referring to using small amounts strategically to help with flavoring or cooking. An example of this would be putting a thin layer of olive oil on your vegetables prior to grilling them.

Rule # 8) Use Sugar Substitutes.

Never go back to using real sugar. Since you have been eating better you have probably noticed that your sweet tooth has diminished. Continue this trend of avoiding things laden in sugar. Keep using fruit to satisfy your sweet tooth. If you need your coffee or tea sweetened, use one of the sugar substitutes. Regular sugar is just concentrated calories that drive up insulin levels, increase the hunger mechanism, and cause weight gain.

Rule # 9) Cook Healthy

Remember to bake, broil, barbeque, boil, grill, and steam your food. Do not fry your foods in oil, butter or animal fat.

Rule # 10) Use Healthy Snacks

This is a good time to begin introducing on occasion some of the healthy cereal and multigrain bars on the market. I want you to remember two things when using these. First, I don't want you to rid your new healthy habit of eating fruit as your snack. Second, many of these bars on the market are as unhealthy as other snack foods. Remember what I said, being healthy will be for the rest of your life. You have to do your homework and research whatever you put in your body.

Many people who follow my diet miss their ice cream. I consider regular ice cream to be the most dangerous food on the market. Not only is it extremely high in fat but also sugar. Once again, I am aware that there are low fat, low carbohydrate ice creams on the market. Similar to cheese, during the weight loss phase, I wanted to rid this taste from your lifestyle and get you in the habit of eating healthier snacks like fruits and yogurts. Now that you have done so, if you desire you can have one of the low fat and carb ice creams on the market, but not the real thing. If you find yourself on vacation with the family and real ice cream is a treat, indulge in it this one time. Don't keep it in your freezer or make this a habit.

Nuts of various varieties, were another snack I prevented you from eating because of their high fat content. Now that the weight is gone, you can reintroduce this natural snack in limited portions.

To summarize the rules of maintenance is not all that difficult. Basically, you will introduce starches cooked in a healthy way. You will bring back some healthy polyunsaturated fats, and can begin to eat some healthy snack foods. Reintroducing these foods will stop the weight loss and if done correctly will prevent weight gain.

The golden rule of maintenance is to weigh yourself everyday.

Now that you have lost the weight that you desired, you have to insure that you never gain it back. To do this will require diligence in following the maintenance rules, along with close observation of your weight. It is very easy to slip into some old habits once you loosen up and start to eat some of the starches and fats once again. Even though you should not gain doing the above, you just might. Weighing yourself once a week was probably adequate while in the weight loss mode, but will not be when you are in the maintenance mode. While in this mode it is absolutely imperative to weigh yourself every single day. While doing this, you will keep your weight within a five pound range. For instance, suppose your goal weight is 147 pounds. While in maintenance you will keep your weight between 145 and 150 pounds. To accomplish this, you will first get your weight to 147 pounds. Once there, you will follow the rules of maintenance and weigh yourself at the same time everyday. I prefer early morning. If your weight stays the same, wonderful, as this is your goal. Often times, you will find yourself straying from your new eating habits and your weight will start to creep up. If you aren't weighing yourself daily, one day you will notice you have gained 15 to 20 pounds or more. Weighing yourself everyday will call attention to any gain early. Since our weight varies a pound or two everyday, it is not enough to be alarmed. However, if you hit that 150 number on the scale, you are going off course. It is at this time you must immediately come out of the maintenance mode and begin to follow the rules and regulations in the weight loss chapters of the book. This time however take yourself down to 145 pounds. It will probably only take 10 to 14 days to lose this 5 pounds, since you have done it before and are now an old pro at it. Once you have hit the 145 mark, restart your maintenance program, this time with a little more leeway. It is crucial to stay in the range of 5 pounds. You may find a few times a year you may have to go into weight loss mode for a week or two but it is a small price to pay. Before I go on vacation, I lose a few pounds before the trip because I know I will be eating in restaurants for all my meals and will tend to gain during these times. The key here is you don't want to find yourself one day behind the eight ball having to start all over again with a lot of weight to lose.

It took a lot of dedication, sacrifice, and a complete change in your thought process and actions to get you to this point. You should be proud of yourself for taking the time to take control of your life and becoming a healthier person. I hope because of it, you will be happier and enjoy life to its fullest potential.

CHAPTER 14

▼

OUTLINES

These outlines will serve as a guideline for you while working on your new way of life. You will notice there is a space between each focus point that comes from the chapters. Use this space for your thoughts. As I mentioned earlier, many people think these writing exercises are useless. I beg to differ. These exercises will help you to visualize your responses on paper. If you look at them regularly, they will not only serve as a constant reminder, they will also be a source for inspiration during times of frustration or when you simply veer off course.

You will also see in this chapter summaries of your rules and regulations for proper eating during your weight loss phase, as well as your maintenance phase.

While trying to lose weight, hang the weight loss outline on your refrigerator to assist you with your food choices. Once your goal weight has been attained, change to the maintenance outline.

You will also see the steps to success repeated. Place these in an area where you can see them daily. Use these steps not only in dieting, but with anything you wish to achieve in your life. They are truly the steps to success and will lead you to your aspirations. In all of these endeavors remember to focus on the end point and enjoy the ride.

Focus points

1) Write down the cost you have paid for your weight

2) Write down the price you will pay without change.

3) Write down the price you will pay to change.

4) Write down what you will ultimately achieve by being your desired weight.

5) Write down your goal weight and date of expectation.

6) Focus on memorizing the 10 rules of weight loss and using your diary to attain your new lifestyle.

7) Never be hungry when you sit down to eat the main meal.

8) Write down how you will accomplish your exercise goals. List ways you will be able to increase your body's activities. Look at these regularly and stick to it faithfully.

9) Write down all of the negative beliefs you have had about yourself in the past and what they have cost you.

10) Write down a new set of positive beliefs and what they will bring to you. Remember to reaffirm them daily.

11) People who are successful with anything in life don't make excuses. When things go wrong, they accept the result, analyze what went wrong, fix it and move on. Do the same with your food habits and your new life.

12) If you stray off your diet or develop resistance, you need to brush it off, and immediately focus on getting back on track.

13) **Link your old habits to your current state of pain and your new habits to your future success.**

14) **Don't focus on your weight, focus on your health and well being.**

15) **In all aspects of life remember the steps for success.**

Steps For Success

1) Reason or Inspiration.

2) Goal or Destination.

3) Belief you can do it.

4) Roadmap on how to get there.

5) Taking Action.

6) Some Sacrifice for the better good.

7) Going through mistakes.

8) Staying focused and perseverance.

9) Attain the final result.

10) Focus on continued success.

Rules and Regulations for weight loss

1) **Lots of Water.** Drink about two quarts a day, especially before meals.

2) **Only Smart Carbohydrates. No sugar, flour, juice, rice, potatoes, or pasta. Cereals** are ok if bran, grain or oat type. No sugar, corn or rice cereals. Oatmeal is fine. **Vegetables** are great, but avoid starchy type vegetables such as corn, carrots, peas, and beats, **Breads** should be wheat or multigrain type and should be sliced or English muffin. No rolls, bagels or other muffins or cake products from dough. **Fruit** should be eaten twice a day as a snack. It means one piece or a small cup and all natural. No canned fruits in any kind of syrup.

3) **Limit Your Fats.** All meat eaten will be low in fat. Turkey, chicken, veal, and fish are perfect. Beef should be filet mignon or sirloin in limited use. Keep away from pork unless rare center cut on rare occasions. No processed meats, unless from chicken or turkey and

specifically states low in fat. This means no hot dogs, sausage, kielbasa, bologna, salami and other processed cold cuts. Low fat types like turkey or chicken burgers or sausage etc, are ok. **No cheese, butter or oil.**

4) No Carbs mixed with Fats. No cake, pastries, cookies, doughnuts, croissants, chips, cheese snacks, chocolate, ice cream etc.

5) No Salt

6) Drink Healthy. Use club soda, flavored waters, diet teas, diet lemonades. Diet soda ok if necessary. No regular soda, beer, wine or hard liquor.

7) Use Healthy Condiments. Use only low fat, low calorie dressings on your salads. **It's ok** to use mustard, ketchup, tobasco sauce, lime or lemon juices, marinades and seasonings, crushed or dried tomatoes, herbs, relish, teriyaki, peppers, salsa, barbeque sauce, sesame, cocktail sauce, peppercorns, garlic, spices, vinegar, Worcestershire, limited margarines and butter sprays. **It's not ok** to use mayonnaise, butter, creamy salad dressings, sour cream, horseradish or tarter sauce, cheese or cheese sauces, oils.

8) Use Sugar Substitutes. Aspartame (Equal), dextrose (Splenda), and saccharin (Sweet n Low) are fine. No regular sugar or even sugar in the raw.

9) Cook Healthy. Bake, broil, grill, roast, barbeque, boil, or steam. Never fry foods in oil, animal fat, or butter. Never fry meat. If frying something else, coat pan lightly with all natural cooking spray like PAM Organic.

10) Always eat snacks or desserts that will help you to your goal. Fruit, diet yogurts, diet puddings, vegetable sticks, cottage cheese.

Sample Diet For Weight Loss

Breakfast:

Cereal made from grain, oats, or wheat, with no more then 3/4 cup of low fat milk up to 3 times a week.
Oatmeal as often as desired cooked in a healthy manner.
Eggbeaters or egg whites. Use no more then 2 eggs, cooked in a pan coated with PAM spray. May use vegetables in omelet if desired. Do not exceed 3 times per week.
Low fat, low carb yogurt or low fat cottage cheese English Muffin. Whole wheat or multigrain type. No more then twice a week

Lunch:

Sandwich Turkey breast, chicken breast, low fat ham, or tuna in water is fine. Use a healthy condiment. A dash of light mayo is acceptable if needed. Use multigrain or whole wheat bread.

Wrap Grilled chicken, shrimp, turkey, tuna, or grilled vegetables are all ok. Use a wheat wrap as opposed to traditional flour wrap.

Soup Use vegetable and chicken soups. No pasta or cream soups.

Salad Use low fat dressing, may add a healthy meat.

Dinner:

Healthy Meat Chicken, turkey, veal, or fish work well. The turkey or chicken may be processed i.e. Burgers, sausage. Fish can be any type. If use steak or beef it must be filet mignon or sirloin and no larger then the hand of an average person.

Vegetable and a salad, or two vegetables should be with every meal.

No starch at the dinner table. No rice, pasta, bread, or potatoes.

Snacks between meals and nighttime ok if are healthy in nature. Use fruits, vegetable sticks, cottage cheese diet yogurts, jello and puddings.

Follow This Pattern For Weight Loss to Avoid Hunger

Healthy Breakfast

Sipping water throughout the morning

Piece of fruit in late morning

Glass of water before lunch

Healthy Lunch

Sip water throughout afternoon

Piece of fruit in late afternoon

Glass of water before dinner

Salad before dinner

Dinner with vegetable

Healthy snack if hungry late night

Rules and Regulations to Maintain Weight

1) Lots of Water

2) Healthy Carbohydrates, may now have healthy starches in moderation. Cook your potatoes, pastas, and rice without the fats.

3) Fats must be polyunsaturated or monounsaturated in limitation.

4) Only smart carbs mixed with healthy fats in limitation

5) Continue to limit salt

6) Continue to drink healthy beverages

7) Continue to use healthy condiments

8) Continue to use sugar substitutes

9) Always cook foods in a healthy manner

10) Use healthy snacks. Try to stick with fruit and yogurts. Healthy cereal or grain bars in moderation can be added

11) THE GOLDEN RULE OF WEIGHT MAIN-TENANCE, IS TO WEIGH YOURSELF EVERY-DAY AND KEEP IT WITHIN A FIVE POUND RANGE.

978-0-595-47778-4
0-595-47778-X

www.ingramcontent.com/pod-product-compliance
Lightning Source LLC
Chambersburg PA
CBHW022232290526
45785CB00014B/724